The Ultimate Lean and Green Cookbook

Kickstart Your Long-Term Transformation| Only Lean, Leaner and Leanest Recipe for Your Selected Plan

By Emily Davis

Copyright - 2020 - All rights reserved.

The content contained within this book may not be reproduced, duplicated or transmitted without direct written permission from the author or the publisher.

Under no circumstances will any blame or legal responsibility be held against the publisher, or author, for any damages, reparation, or monetary loss due to the information contained within this book. Either directly or indirectly.

Legal Notice:

This book is copyright protected. This book is only for personal use. You cannot amend, distribute, sell, use, quote or paraphrase any part, or the content within this book, without the consent of the author or publisher.

Disclaimer Notice:

Please note the information contained within this document is for educational and entertainment purpose sonly. All effort has been executed to present accurate, upto date, and reliable, complete information. No warranties of any kind are declared or implied. Readers acknowledge that the author is not engaging in the rendering of legal, financial, medical or professional advice. The content within this book has been derived from various sources. Please consult a licensed professional before attempting any techniques outlined in this book. By reading this document, the reader agrees that under no circumstances is the author responsible for any losses, direct or indirect, which are incurred as a result of the use of information contained within this document, including, but not limited to, - errors, omissions, or inaccuracies.

1. Introduction 7
2. Lean And Green Recipe 8
    1) Healthy Peppers Flounder MeatBall 9
    2) A Triumph of Meat and Vegetables 9
    3) Garlic and Oil – Broccoli and Beef 9
    4) Meat in he Woods 10
    5) Turkey on Boat 10
    6) Wedding of Broccoli and Tomatoes 10
    7) Hamburger Salad 10
    8) Green Buddha Smile 11
    9) Zucchini Fettuccine with Mexican Taco 11
    10) Onion Green Beans 11
    11) Cream Of Mushroom Satay 12
    12) Tortoreto Mushrooms with Ceddar 12
    13) Chicken Goulash with Green Peppers 13
    14) Lettuce Salad with Beef Strips 13
    15) Cauliflower Sprinkled with Curry 13
    16) Pork Stew with Green Chili 14
    17) Coriander Spice Salmon 14
    18) Roast Beef Greek Recipe 15
    19) Tomatoes in The Mushroom 15
    20) Shrimp Cocktails with Tomato and Lettuce 16
    21) Celeriac Mix with Cauliflower 16
    22) Cheddar Fondue with Tomato Sauce 16
    23) Baked Salmon Garnished with Mustard 17
    24) Quick Spinach Focaccia 17
    25) Sizzling Chicken Salad 18
    26) Italian-Style Seasoned Fish Fillet 18
    27) Triumph of Cucumbers and Avocado 18
    28) Salmon Burger With Broccoli 18
    29) Tuna Focaccia 19
    30) Delicious Tomato Broth 19
    31) Baked Salmon Souffle 19
    32) Spinach and Tomato Omelette 19
    33) Vegan Turkey 19
    34) Fettuccine with Turkey Ragù 20
    35) Smoked Range Chicken 20
    36) Earl Ground Beef 21
    37) A Cup of Cauliflower Taco 22
    38) Prawn Broccoli 22
    39) Creamy Mushroom Tornado 22
    40) Boscaiola Beef Fillet 23
    41) Bed of Mushroom with Stir-Fried Tofu 23
    42) Turkey Sesame Scent 23
    43) Lime-Mint Soup 24
    44) Brussels Sprouts Stew 25
    45) Tomato Pumpkin Soup 25
    46) Creamy Squash Soup 25
    47) Sautéed Collard greens 26
    48) Spinach Soup with Dill and Basil 26
    49) Cream of Mushroom Soup 26
    50) Coconut Watercress Soup 27
    51) Creamy Celery Soup 27
    52) Cajun Sweet Potatoes 27
    53) Mediterranean Hummus Pizza 28
    54) Turnip Chips 28
    55) Miso Spaghetti Squash 28
    56) Tortilla Chips 29
    57) Navy Beans, Spinach, and Artichoke Spread 29
    58) Broccoli Salad with Cheese 29
    59) Pea Salad 30
3. Quick and Easy Recipe for Busy Worker 32
    60) Salted Cod Lemon 33

- 61) Flounder Lemon Sauce 33
- 62) Scallop Sauce With Butter and Garlic 33
- 63) Baltic Tacos 34
- 64) Garlic Green Beans Sautéed with Parmesan 34
- 65) Paprika Pork in Garlic Sauce 34
- 66) Chicken Stuffed with Cauliflower 35
- 67) Spicy Mushroom Collard Wraps 35
- 68) Tofu Scalloppini & Lemon 36
- 69) Creamy Fettuccine with Peas 36
- 70) Broccoli Salad with Cheese 37
- 71) Creamy Cauliflower Chipotle Spread 37
- 72) Red Potatoes and Green Beans 37
- 73) Green Beans Side Salad 38
- 74) Corn Bread 38
- 75) Smoky Coleslaw 38
- 76) Vegan Chocolate Orange Truffles 39
- 77) Broccoli Salad 39
- 78) Zucchini Pasta Salad 39
- 79) Polenta with Pears and Cranberries 39

4. Fuelings Recipe 40

- 80) Light Chocolate Bars 41
- 81) Mexican Pudding 41
- 82) Brazilian Pudding 41
- 83) Peanut Butter Delight 41
- 84) Raspberry Ice Cream 41
- 85) Chocolate Almond Bites 42
- 86) Butter Creamy Fudge 42
- 87) Cocoa Chocolate Mousse 42
- 88) Almond Bites 42
- 89) Coffe Blend Mousse 42
- 90) Light Cake 43
- 91) Cinnamon Explosion 43
- 92) Greek Breakfast 43
- 93) Diet Tomato Cookies 44
- 94) Diet Haystacks 44
- 95) Cheesecake Cookies 44
- 96) Borough Eggs 44
- 97) Tasty Diet Lemon Meringue 45
- 98) Peanut Butter Crunch Bars 45
- 99) Grilled Cheese Tomato Sandwich 45
- 100) Faux Fried Zucchini 46
- 101) Chocolate Mint Soft Serve Brownie Bottoms . 46
- 102) Slutty Brownie 46
- 103) Chocolate Chip Cakes 46
- 104) Pistachio Shake 47
- 105) Pudding Pies 47
- 106) Chocolate Cheesecake Shake 47

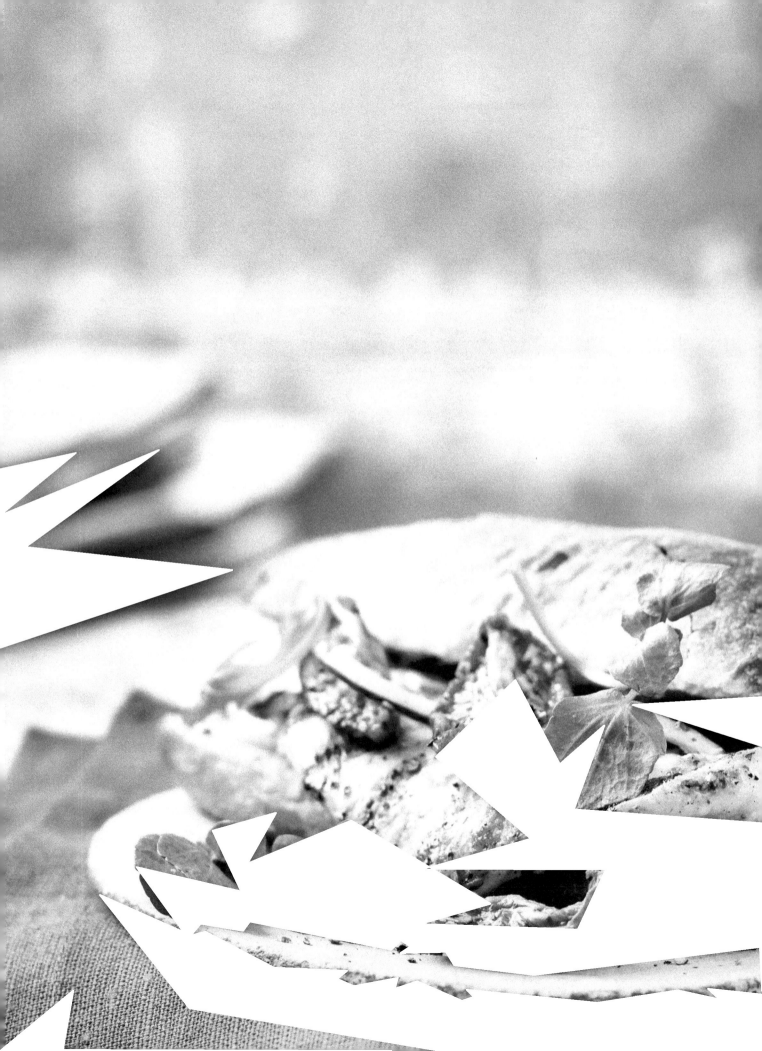

1. Introduction

How hard is, following a diet!

No one knows more than me how hard can be to try a new path like dieting, trying again and again to change your habits and constantly FAIL!

But...wow! You're stronger than me, you decided to take antother path!

The diet you decided to approach has nothing to do with traditional diets, as ketogenic, atkins or plant-based diet.

Look at the points in its favour:

- *You can decide how to manage meals and meal times*
- *You're supported by a coach that approached the same path as you, before you started. She knows about it every aspect, good and bad times, joys and pains. Who better than her/him can guide you in such a path and help you to rich your goals in the best way?*

You're wondering at this point why this book was created

Let's first of all look at the reasons why it is NOT created:

- *It was not born to explain the advantages or disadvantages of following the path you've taken*
- *It was not born to explain the differences between the various feeding plans*
- *It was not born to teach you a food plan thrown in at random*
- *It was not born to give you confusing recipes, or not relevant with the path you decided together with your coach*

This book was created to give you all the recipes you need to complete the path you decided with your coach

You'll have to eat at least one of these meals a day during your path

Avoid always eating the same things and take inspiration from my recipes

Each recipe respects the directive (Lean, Leanest, Leaner)

Always bring it with you, crumple it, stain it...use it!

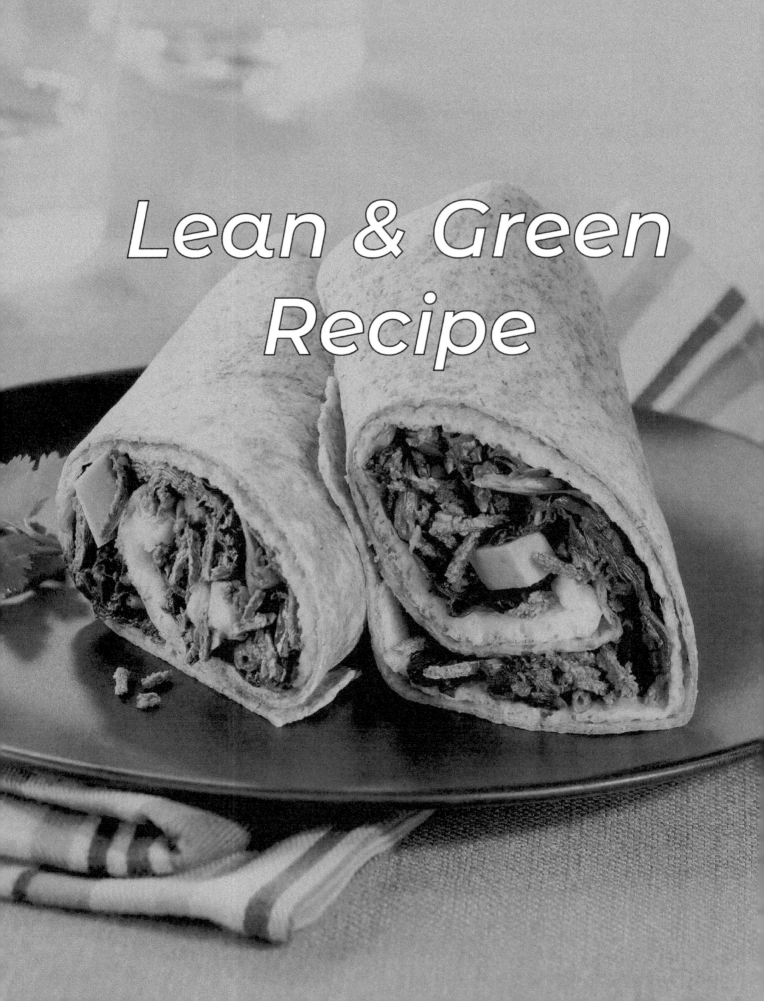

1) Healthy Peppers Flounder MeatBall

Serves: 3

Cooking Time: 6 minutes

Nutrition: Calories per serving: 380; Protein: 28.7g; Carbs: 13g; Fat: 5.4g Sugar: 0.02g

Leanest Recipe

Ingredients:
- 10 ounces flounder fillet, chopped finely
- 1/3 cup celery stalk, chopped finely
- 1/3 cup red pepper, chopped finely
- 1 tablespoon fresh dill, chopped finely
- 2 teaspoons Dijon mustard
- 2 eggs, slightly beaten
- Salt and pepper to taste

Directions:
1. Place all ingredients in a bowl. Mix until well-incorporated.
2. Form small patties with your hands and place on a baking sheet. Allow patties to rest in the fridge for at least 30
3. minutes.
4. Brush pan with extra virgin olive oil and allow to heat over medium flame.
5. Place individual patties into the pan and cook for 3 minutes on each side.
6. Serve immediately.

2) A Triumph of Meat and Vegetables

Serves: 3

Cooking Time: 10 minutes

Nutrition: Calories per serving: 174; Protein: 4.2g; Carbs: 10.3g; Fat: 4.1g Sugar: 2.1g

Leaner Recipe

Ingredients:
- 1/2 teaspoon extra virgin olive oil
- 2 ounces Sirloin steak, 98% lean
- Salt and pepper to taste
- 1 zucchini, cut into long thin strips
- 1 onion, chopped
- 6 ounces asparagus, blanched
- 4 ounces peas, blanched

Directions:
1. Heat olive oil in a skillet. Season the steak with salt and pepper to taste.
2. Place in the skillet and sear the steak for 5 minutes on each side. Allow to rest for five minutes before slicing into strips.
3. Place the remaining ingredients in a bowl and season with salt and pepper to taste
4. Top with steak strips then toss to combine all ingredients.

3) Garlic and Oil – Broccoli and Beef

Serves: 4

Cooking Time: 15 minutes

Nutrition: Calories per serving: 186; Protein: 21g; Carbs: 8.7g; Fat: 3.1g Sugar: 0.8g

Lean Recipe

Ingredients:
- 4 ounces 95-97% lean ground beef
- 1/4 cup roma tomatoes, chopped
- 1/4 teaspoon garlic powder
- 1/4 teaspoon onion powder
- 1 1/4 cup broccoli, cut into bite-sized pieces
- A pinch of red pepper flakes
- 1 ounce low-sodium cheddar cheese, shredded

Directions:
1. Place 3 tablespoons of water in a pan and heat over medium flame.
2. Water sauté the beef and tomatoes for 5 minutes until the tomatoes are wilted. Add in the garlic and onion powder and stir for another 3 minutes.
3. Add the broccoli and close the lid. Cook for another 5 minutes.
4. Garnish with red pepper flakes and cheddar cheese on top.

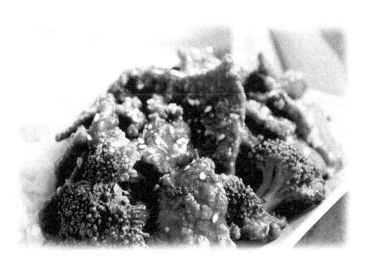

4) Meat in he Woods

Serves: 6

Cooking Time: 7 minutes

Nutrition: Calories per serving: 186; Protein: 21g; Carbs: 8.7g; Fat: 3.1g Sugar: 0.8g

Lean Recipe

Ingredients:
- 1 pound 98% lean ground beef
- A pinch of salt
- 1/4 teaspoon black pepper
- 8 ounces Romaine lettuce, torn
- 1 cup cherry tomatoes, halved
- 1/2 cup pickles, diced
- 1/4 cup cheddar cheese, shredded

Directions:
1. Season the beef with salt and pepper.
2. Heat a non-stick pan and sauté the beef white stirring constantly for 7 minutes. Set aside and allow to slightly
3. cool.
4. Place the lettuce, tomatoes, pickles, and cheese. Sprinkle the cooked beef on top.
5. Toss to mix all ingredients.

5) Turkey on Boat

Serves: 8

Cooking Time: 20 minutes

Nutrition: Calories per serving: 115; Protein: 13.2g; Carbs: 6.3g; Fat: 1.4g Sugar: 0.5g

Leaner recipe

Ingredients:
- 4 medium zucchinis
- 2 tablespoons extra virgin olive oil
- 1-pound lean ground turkey
- 3 cloves of garlic, minced
- 1/2 onion, chopped
- 1/2 green pepper, seeded and chopped
- 1/2 cup skimmed mozzarella cheese, shredded

Directions:
1. Prepare the zucchini by slicing them in half lengthwise. Scoop the meat out. Chopped the scooped-up zucchini meat and set aside.
2. Heat oil in a saucepan over medium flame. Stir in the turkey and garlic and sauté for 5 minutes.
3. Stir in the onions halfway while the turkey is cooking. Add in the green pepper and zucchini meat. Cook for
4. another 3 minutes. Set aside to cool completely.
5. Once cooled, stir in the mozzarella cheese.
6. Fill the hollowed-out zucchini with the meat mixture.
7. Place in a 3600F preheated oven and bake for 10 minutes.

6) Wedding of Broccoli and Tomatoes

Serves: 3

Cooking Time: 2 minutes

Nutrition: Calories per serving: 52; Protein: 1.1g; Carbs: 3.2g; Fat: 0.1g Sugar: 0.2g

Leanest recipe

Ingredients:
- 1 head broccoli, cut into florets then blanched
- 1/4 cup tomatoes, diced
- Salt and pepper to taste
- Chopped parsley for garnish

Directions:
- Place all ingredients in a bowl.
- Toss to coat all ingredients.
- 3. Serve.

7) Hamburger Salad

Serves: 6

Cooking Time: 7 minutes

Nutrition: Calories per serving: 186; Protein: 21g; Carbs: 8.7g; Fat: 3.1g Sugar: 0.8g

Lean Recipe

Ingredients:
- 1 pound 98% lean ground beef
- A pinch of salt
- 1/4 teaspoon black pepper
- 8 ounces Romaine lettuce, torn
- 1 cup cherry tomatoes, halved
- 1/2 cup pickles, diced
- 1/4 cup cheddar cheese, shredded

Directions:
1. Season the beef with salt and pepper.
2. Heat a non-stick pan and sauté the beef white stirring constantly for 7 minutes. Set aside and allow to slightly cool.
3. Place the lettuce, tomatoes, pickles, and cheese. Sprinkle the cooked beef on top.
4. Toss to mix all ingredients.

8) *Green Buddha Smile*

Serves: 6

Cooking Time: 10 minutes

Nutrition: Calories total: 411; Protein: 44.2g; Carbs: 40.4g; Fat: 4g Sugar: 3g

Leaner recipe

Ingredients:
- 2 pounds boneless and skinless chicken breast
- 2 tablespoons lemon juice, freshly squeezed
- Salt and pepper to taste
- 1-pound Brussels sprouts, trimmed and halved
- 3 cloves of garlic, minced
- 3/4 cup plain Greek yogurt
- 1 teaspoon stone-ground mustard
- 1/4 cup balsamic vinegar
- 2 cups cooked quinoa
- 1 cup chopped red apple, cored, and chopped
- 1/4 cup pepitas
- 1 avocado, sliced
- 1 1/2 cup arugula
- 1 tablespoon fresh basil

Directions:
1. Place chicken and lemon juice in a bowl. Season with salt and pepper to taste. Allow to marinate in the fridge for at least 30 minutes.
2. Fire up the grill to 3750F and cook the chicken for 6 minutes on each side. Add in the Brussels sprouts and cook for 3 minutes on each side. Set the chicken and Brussels sprouts aside.
3. In a bowl, mix together the garlic, yogurt, mustard, and vinegar. Season with salt to taste. Set aside.
4. On a bowl, place the quinoa and top with apple, pepitas, avocado, and arugula. Top with grilled chicken and Brussels sprouts.
5. Drizzle with the sauce and garnish with basil.

9) *Zucchini Fettuccine with Mexican Taco*

Serves: 6

Cooking Time: 20 minutes

Nutrition: Calories per serving: 145; Protein: 15g; Carbs: 8.5g; Fat:2.1 g Sugar: 0.5g

Leaner recipe

Ingredients:
- 1 tablespoon olive oil
- 1-pound lean ground turkey
- 1 clove garlic, minced
- 1/2 small onion, chopped
- 1 tablespoon chili powder
- 1/4 teaspoon garlic powder
- 1/4 teaspoon onion powder
- 1/4 teaspoon dried oregano
- 1 1/2 teaspoon ground cumin
- 1/4 cup water
- 1/4 cup diced tomatoes
- 2 large zucchinis, spiralized
- 1/2 cup shredded cheddar cheese

Directions:
1. Place oil in a pot and heat over medium flame.
2. Sauté the turkey for 2 minutes before adding the garlic and onions. Stir for another minute.
3. Season with chili powder, garlic powder, onion powder, oregano, and ground cumin. Sauté for another minute
4. before adding the water and tomatoes.
5. Close the lid and allow to simmer for 7 minutes.
6. Add in the zucchini and cheese and allow to cook for 3 more minutes.

10) *Onion Green Beans*

Serves: 2

Cooking time: 12 minutes

Nutrition: Calories total: 302 Fat: 7.2g Fiber: 5.5g Carbohydrates: 13.9g Protein: 3.2g

Leanest recipe

Ingredients:
- 11 oz. green beans
- 1 tablespoon of onion powder 1 tablespoon of olive oil
- 1/2 teaspoon of salt
- 1/4 teaspoon of red pepper flakes

Directions:
1. Wash the green beans thoroughly and put them in the bowl.
2. Sprinkle the green beans with lion's powder, salt, chillies, and olive oil.
3. Shake the green bean carefully.
4. Preheat the 400F air refrigerator.
5. Place the green beans in the deep fryer and cook for 8 minutes.
6. Next, shake the green beans and cook them for 4 minutes or more at 400 F. 7. When time remains: shake the green beans.
7. Serve them with joy!

11) Cream Of Mushroom Satay

Serves: 2

Cooking Time: 6 minutes

Nutrition: Calories per serving: 116 Fat: 9.5g Fiber: 1.3g Carbs: 5.6g Protein: 3g

Leanest recipe

Ingredients:
- 7 oz. cremini mushrooms
- 2 tablespoon coconut milk
- 1 tablespoon butter
- 1 teaspoon chili flakes
- ½ teaspoon balsamic vinegar
- ½ teaspoon curry powder
- ½ teaspoon white pepper

Directions:
1. Wash the mushrooms carefully.
2. Then sprinkle the mushrooms with the chili flakes, curry powder, and white pepper.
3. Preheat the air fryer to 400 F.
4. Toss the butter in the air fryer basket and melt it.
5. Put the mushrooms in the air fryer and cook for 2 minutes.
6. Shake the mushrooms well and sprinkle with the coconut milk and balsamic vinegar.
7. Cook the mushrooms for 4 minutes more at 400 F.
8. Then skewer the mushrooms on the wooden sticks and serve.
9. Enjoy!

12) Tortoreto Mushrooms with Ceddar

Serves: 2

Cooking Time: 6 minutes

Nutrition: Calories total: 376 Fat: 24.1g Fiber: 1.8g Carbs: 14.6g Protein: 25.2g

Leanest recipe

Ingredients:
- 2 Tortoreto mushroom hats
- 2 slices Cheddar cheese
- ¼ cup panko breadcrumbs
- ½ teaspoon salt
- ½ teaspoon ground black pepper
- 1 egg
- 1 teaspoon oatmeal
- 2 oz. bacon, chopped cooked

Directions:
1. Crack the egg into the bowl and whisk it.
2. Combine the ground black pepper, oatmeal, salt, and breadcrumbs in the separate bowl.
3. Dip the mushroom hats in the whisked egg.
4. After this, coat the mushroom hats in the breadcrumb mixture.
5. Preheat the air fryer to 400 F.
6. Place the mushrooms in the air fryer basket tray and cook for 3 minutes.
7. After this, put the chopped bacon and sliced cheese over the mushroom hats and cook the meal for 3 minutes.
8. When the meal is cooked – let it chill gently.
9. Enjoy!

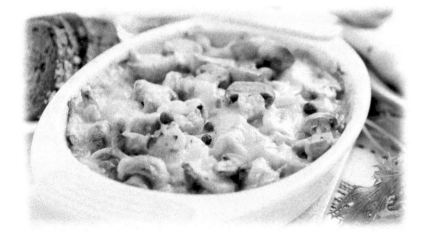

13) *Chicken Goulash with Green Peppers*

Serves: 6

Cooking Time: 17 minutes

Nutrition: Calories per serving: 161 Fat: 6.1g Carbs: 6g Protein: 20.3g

Leaner Recipe

Ingredients:
- 4 oz. chive stems
- 2 green peppers, chopped
- 1 teaspoon olive oil
- 14 oz. ground chicken
- 2 tomatoes
- ½ cup chicken stock
- 2 garlic cloves, sliced
- 1 teaspoon salt
- 1 teaspoon ground black pepper
- 1 teaspoon mustard

Directions:
1. Chop chives roughly.
2. Spray the air fryer basket tray with the olive oil.
3. Preheat the air fryer to 365 F.
4. Put the chopped chives in the air fryer basket tray.
5. Add the chopped green pepper and cook the vegetables for 5 minutes.
6. Add the ground chicken.
7. Chop the tomatoes into the small cubes and add them in the air fryer mixture too.
8. Cook the mixture for 6 minutes more.
9. Add the chicken stock, sliced garlic cloves, salt, ground black pepper, and mustard.
10. Mix well to combine.
11. Cook the goulash for 6 minutes more.

14) *Lettuce Salad with Beef Strips*

Serves: 5

Cooking Time: 12 minutes

Nutrition: Calories per serving: 199 Fat: 12.4g Carbs: 3.9g Protein: 18.1g

Lean Recipe

Ingredients:
- 2 cup lettuce
- 10 oz. beef brisket
- 2 tablespoon sesame oil
- 1 tablespoon sunflower seeds
- 1 cucumber
- 1 teaspoon ground black pepper
- 1 teaspoon paprika
- 1 teaspoon Italian spices
- 2 teaspoon butter
- 1 teaspoon dried dill
- 2 tablespoon coconut milk

Directions:
1. Cut the beef brisket into strips. Sprinkle the beef strips with the ground black pepper, paprika, and dried dill.
2. Preheat the air fryer to 365 F. Put the butter in the air fryer basket tray and melt it.
3. Then add the beef strips and cook them for 6 minutes on each side. Meanwhile, tear the lettuce and toss it in a big salad bowl.
4. Crush the sunflower seeds and sprinkle over the lettuce.
5. Chop the cucumber into the small cubes and add to the salad bowl.
6. Then combine the sesame oil and Italian spices together. Stir the oil.
7. Combine the lettuce mixture with the coconut milk and stir it using 2 wooden spatulas. When the meat is cooked – let it chill to room temperature.
8. Add the beef strips to the salad bowl.
9. Stir it gently and sprinkle the salad with the sesame oil dressing.
10. Serve the dish immediately.

15) *Cauliflower Sprinkled with Curry*

Serves: 4

Cooking Time: 5 hours

Nutrition: Calories per serving: 160 Fat: 11.5g Fiber: 5.4g Carbs: 14.7g Protein: 3.6g

Leanest Recipe

Ingredients:
- 1 cauliflower head, florets separated
- 2 carrots, sliced
- 1 red onion, chopped
- ¾ cup coconut milk
- 2 garlic cloves, minced
- 2 tablespoons curry powder
- A pinch of salt and black pepper
- 1 tablespoon red pepper flakes
- 1 teaspoon garam masala

Directions:
1. In your slow cooker, mix all the ingredients.
2. Cover, cook on high for 5 hours, divide into bowls and serve.

16) *Pork Stew with Green Chili*

Serves: 4

Cooking Time: 20 minutes

Nutrition: Calories total: 370 Protein: 36g Carbohydrate: 14g Fat: 19 g

Leaner Recipe

Ingredients:
- 2 scallions, chopped
- 2 cloves of garlic
- 1 lb. tomatillos, trimmed and chopped
- 8 large romaine or green lettuce leaves, divided
- 2 serrano chilies, seeds, and membranes
- ½ tsp of dried Mexican oregano (or you can use regular oregano)
- 1 ½ lb. of boneless pork loin, to be cut into bite-sized cubes
- ¼ cup of cilantro, chopped
- ¼ tablespoon (each) salt and paper
- 1 jalapeno, seeds and membranes to be removed and thinly sliced
- 1 cup of sliced radishes
- 4 lime wedges

Directions:
1. Combine scallions, garlic, tomatillos, 4 lettuce leaves, serrano chilies, and oregano in a blender. Then puree until smooth
2. Put pork and tomatillo mixture in a medium pot. 1-inch of puree should cover the pork; if not, add water until it covers it. Season with pepper & salt, and cover it simmers. Simmer on heat for approximately 20 minutes.
3. Now, finely shred the remaining lettuce leaves.
4. When the stew is done cooking, garnish with cilantro, radishes, finely shredded lettuce, sliced jalapenos, and lime wedges.

17) *Coriander Spice Salmon*

Serves: 4

Cooking Time: 30 minutes

Nutrition: Calories total: 350 Carbohydrate: 15 g Protein: 42 g Fat: 13 g

Lean Recipe

Ingredients:
- 2 tablespoons of fresh lime or lemon
- 4 cups of fresh cilantro, divided
- 2 tablespoon of hot red pepper sauce
- ½ teaspoon of salt. Divided
- 1 teaspoon of cumin
- 4, 7 oz. of salmon filets
- ½ cup of (4 oz.) water
- 2 cups of sliced red bell pepper
- 2 cups of sliced yellow bell pepper
- 2 cups of sliced green bell pepper
- Cooking spray
- ½ teaspoon of pepper

Directions:
1. Get a blender or food processor and combine half of the cilantro, lime juice or lemon, cumin, hot red pepper sauce, water, and salt; then puree until they become smooth. Transfer the marinade gotten into a large re-sealable plastic bag.
2. Add salmon to marinade. Seal the bag, squeeze out air that might have been trapped inside, turn to coat salmon. Refrigerate for about 1 hour, turning as often as possible.
3. Now, after marinating, preheat your oven to about 400°F. Arrange the pepper slices in a single layer in a slightly-greased, medium-sized square baking dish. Bake it for 20 minutes, turn the pepper slices once.
4. Drain your salmon and do away with the marinade. Crust the upper part of the salmon with the remaining chopped, fresh cilantro. Place salmon on the top of the pepper slices and bake for about 12-14 minutes until you observe that the fish flakes easily when it is being tested with a fork
5. Enjoy

18) Roast Beef Greek Recipe

Cooking Time: 8 hours

Nutrition: Calories per serving: 231 Fat: 6 g Carbohydrates: 4 g Sugar: 1.4 g Protein: 35 g Cholesterol: 75 mg

Lean Recipe

- 2 lbs lean top round beef roast
- 1 tablespoon Italian seasoning
- 6 garlic cloves, minced
- 1 onion, sliced
- 2 cups beef broth
- ½ cup red wine
- 1 teaspoon red pepper flakes
- Pepper
- Salt

1. Season meat with pepper and salt and place into the crock pot.
2. Pour remaining ingredients over meat.
3. Cover and cook on low heat for 8 hours.
4. Shred the meat using fork.
5. Serve and enjoy.

Serves: 4

Cooking time: 50 minutes

Nutrition: Calories per serving: 160 Carbs: 2 g Fat: 11 g Protein: 4 g Fiber: 0 g

Leaner Recipe

edients:
- 8 large mushrooms
- 250g of minced meat
- 4 cloves of garlic
- Extra virgin olive oil
- Salt
- Ground pepper
- Flour, beaten egg and breadcrumb
- Frying oil
- Fried Tomato Sauce

Directions:
1. Remove the stem from the mushrooms and chop it. Peel the garlic and chop. Put some extra virgin olive oil in a pan and add the garlic and mushroom stems.
2. Sauté and add the minced meat. Sauté well until the meat is well cooked and season.
3. Fill the mushrooms with the minced meat.
4. Press well and take the freezer for 30 minutes.
5. Pass the mushrooms with flour, beaten egg and breadcrumbs. Beaten egg and breadcrumbs.
6. Place the mushrooms in the basket of the air fryer.
7. Select 20 minutes, 180°C (350°F).
8. Distribute the mushrooms once cooked in the dishes.
9. Heat the tomato sauce and cover the stuffed mushrooms.

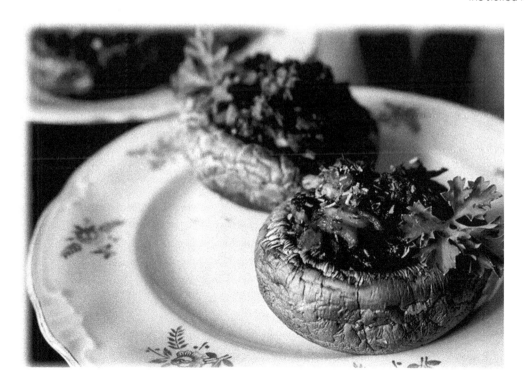

20) *Shrimp Cocktails with Tomato and Lettuce*

Serves: 8 Serves

Cooking Time: 35 minutes

Nutrition Information:

Calories total: 580 Total Carbohydrate: 16 g Cholesterol: 192 mg Total Fat: 46 g Fiber: 2 g Protein: 24 g

Leanest Recipe

Ingredients:
- 2 cups mayonnaise
- 6 plum tomatoes, seeded and finely chopped
- 1/4 cup ketchup
- 1/4 cup lemon juice
- 2 cups seedless red and/or green grapes, halved
- 1 tablespoon. Worcestershire sauce
- 2 lbs. peeled and deveined cooked large shrimp
- 2 celery ribs, finely chopped
- 3 tablespoons. minced fresh tarragon or 3 teaspoon dried tarragon
- salt and 1/4 teaspoon pepper
- shredded 2 of cups romaine
- papaya or 1/2 cup peeled chopped mango
- parsley or minced chives

Directions:
1. Combine Worcestershire sauce, lemon juice, ketchup and mayonnaise together in a small bowl.
2. Combine pepper, salt, tarragon, celery and shrimp together in a large bowl.
3. Put in 1 cup of dressing toss well to coat.
4. Scoop 1 tablespoon of the dressing into 8 cocktail glasses.
5. Layer each glass with 1/4 cup of lettuce, followed by 1/2 cup of the shrimp mixture, 1/4 cup of grapes, 1/3 cup of tomatoes and finally 1 tablespoon of mango.
6. Spread the remaining dressing over top; sprinkle chives on top.
7. Serve immediately.

21) *Celeriac Mix with Cauliflower*

Serves: 6

Cooking Time: 12 minutes

Nutrition Information: Calories per serving: 225 Total Carbohydrate: 4 g Cholesterol: 1 mg Total Fat: 20 g Fiber: 0 g Protein: 5 g

Leanest Recipe

Ingredients:
- 1 head cauliflower
- 1 small celery root
- 1/4 cup butter
- 1 tablespoon. chopped rosemary
- 1 tablespoon. chopped thyme
- 1 cup cream cheese

Directions:
1. Skin the celery root and cut into small pieces.
2. Cut the cauliflower into similar sized pieces and combine.
3. Toast the herbs in the butter in a large pan, until they become fragrant.
4. Add the cauliflower and celery root and stir to combine.
5. Season and cook at medium high until whatever moisture is in the vegetables releases itself, then covers and cook on low for 10-12 minutes.
6. Once the vegetables are soft, remove from the heat and place them in the blender.
7. Make it smooth, then put the cream cheese and puree again.
8. Season and serve.

22) *Cheddar Fondue with Tomato Sauce*

Serves: 3-1/2 cups

Cooking Time: 30 minutes

Nutrition: Calories per serving: 118 Total Carbohydrate: 4 g Cholesterol: 30 mg Total Fat: 10 g Fiber: 1 g Protein: 4 g

Leanest Recipe

Ingredients:
- 1 garlic clove, halved
- 6 medium tomatoes, seeded and diced
- 2/3 cup dry white wine
- 6 tablespoons. Butter, cubed
- 1-1/2 teaspoons. Dried basil
- Dash cayenne pepper
- 2 cups shredded cheddar cheese
- 1 tablespoon. All-purpose flour
- Cubed French bread and cooked shrimp

Directions:
1. Rub the bottom and sides of a fondue pot with a garlic clove.
2. Set aside and discard the garlic.
3. Combine wine, butter, basil, cayenne and tomatoes in a large saucepan.
4. On a medium low heat, bring mixture to a simmer, then decrease heat to low.
5. Mix cheese with flour.
6. Add to tomato mixture gradually while stirring after each addition until cheese is melted.
7. Pour into the Preparation timeared fondue pot and keep warm.
8. Enjoy with shrimp and bread cubes.

23) *Baked Salmon Garnished with Mustard*

Serves: 5

Cooking Time: 30 minutes

Nutrition: Calories per serving: 217 Fat 11 g Carbs 2 g Sugar 0.2 g Protein 27 g Cholesterol 60 mg

Lean Recipe

Ingredients:
- 1 1/2 lbs salmon
- 1/4 cup Dijon mustard
- 1/4 cup fresh parsley, chopped
- 1 tbsp garlic, chopped
- 1 tbsp olive oil
- 1 tbsp fresh lemon juice
- Pepper
- Salt

Directions:
1. Preheat the oven to 375 F. Line baking sheet with parchment paper.
2. Arrange salmon fillets on a prepared baking sheet.
3. In a small bowl, mix together garlic, oil, lemon juice, Dijon mustard, parsley, pepper, and salt.
4. Brush salmon top with garlic mixture.
5. Bake for 18-20 minutes.
6. Serve and enjoy.

24) *Quick Spinach Focaccia*

Serves: 12

Cooking Time: 25 minutes

Nutrition: Calories per serving 110 Fat 7 g Carbs 1 g Sugar 0.3 g Protein 9 g Cholesterol 165 mg

Leanest Recipe

Ingredients:
- 10 eggs
- 2 cups spinach, chopped
- 1/4 tsp garlic powder
- 1/4 tsp onion powder
- 1/2 tsp dried basil
- 1 1/2 cups parmesan cheese, grated
- Salt

Directions:
1. Preheat the oven to 400 F. Grease muffin tin and set aside.
2. In a large bowl, whisk eggs with basil, garlic powder, onion powder, and salt.
3. Add cheese and spinach and stir well.
4. Pour egg mixture into the prepared muffin tin and bake 15 minutes.
5. Serve and enjoy.

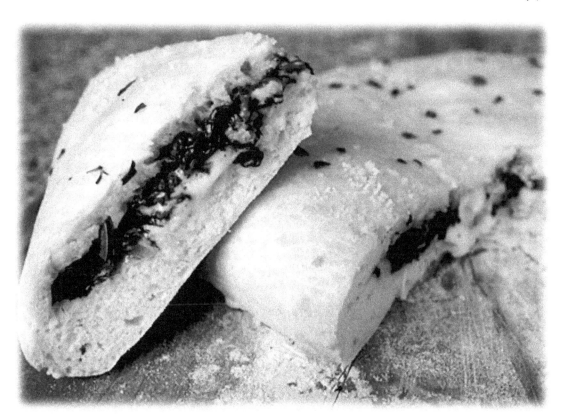

25) *Sizzling Chicken Salad*

Serves: 4

Cooking Time: 15 minutes

Calories total: 172 Fat 7.9 g Carbs 6.7 g Sugar 3.1 g Protein 18.1 g Cholesterol 52 mg

Leaner Recipe

Ingredients:
- 1 1/2 cups chicken breast, skinless, boneless, and cooked
- 2 tbsp onion, diced
- 1/4 cup olives, diced
- 1/4 cup roasted red peppers, diced
- 1/4 cup cucumbers, diced
- 1/4 cup celery, diced
- 1/4 cup feta cheese, crumbled
- 1/2 tsp onion powder
- 1/2 tbsp fresh lemon juice
- 1 tbsp fresh parsley, chopped
- 1 tbsp fresh dill, chopped
- 2 1/2 tbsp mayonnaise
- 1/4 cup Greek yogurt
- 1/4 tsp pepper
- 1/2 tsp salt

Directions:
1. In a bowl, mix together yogurt, onion powder, lemon juice, parsley, dill, mayonnaise, pepper, and salt.
2. Add chicken, onion, olives, red peppers, cucumbers, and feta cheese and stir well.
3. Serve and enjoy.

26) *Italian-Style Seasoned Fish Fillet*

Serves: 1

Cooking Time: 40 minutes

Nutrition: Calories per serving: 383 Fat 22.5 g Carbs 0.8 g Sugar 0.6 g Protein 46.5 g Cholesterol 2 mg

Leanest Recipe

Ingredients:
- 8 oz frozen white fish fillet
- 1 tbsp roasted red bell pepper, diced
- 1/2 tsp Italian seasoning
- 1 tbsp fresh parsley, chopped
- 1 1/2 tbsp olive oil
- 1 tbsp lemon juice

Directions:
- Preheat the oven to 400 F. Line baking sheet with foil.
- Place a fish fillet on a baking sheet.
- Drizzle oil and lemon juice over fish. Season with Italian seasoning.
- Top with roasted bell pepper and parsley and bake for 30 minutes.
- Serve and enjoy.

27) *Triumph of Cucumbers and Avocado*

Serves: 4

Cooking Time: 15 minutes

Nutrition: Calories total: 442 Fat 37.1 g Carbs 30.3 g Sugar 9.4 g Protein 6.2 g Cholesterol 0

Leanest Recipe

Ingredients:
- 12 oz cherry tomatoes, cut in half
- 5 small cucumbers, chopped
- 3 small avocados, chopped
- 1/2 tsp ground black pepper
- 2 tbsp olive oil
- 2 tbsp fresh lemon juice
- 1/4 cup fresh cilantro, chopped
- 1 tsp sea salt

Directions:
1. Add cherry tomatoes, cucumbers, avocados, and cilantro into the large mixing bowl and mix well.
2. Mix together olive oil, lemon juice, black pepper, and salt and pour over salad.
3. Toss well and serve immediately.

28) *Salmon Burger With Broccoli*

Serves: 5

Cooking Time: 30 minutes

Nutrition: Calories per serving: 221 Fat 12.6 g Carbs 5.2 g Sugar 1.4 g Protein 22.1 g Cholesterol 112 mg

Lean Recipe

Ingredients:
- 2 eggs
- 1/2 cup onion, chopped
- 1/2 cup broccoli, chopped
- 1/2 cup kale, chopped
- 1/2 tsp garlic powder
- 2 tbsp lemon juice
- 1/2 cup almond flour
- 15 oz can salmon, drained and bones removed
- 1/2 tsp salt

Directions:
1. Line one plate with parchment paper and set aside.
2. Add all ingredients into the large bowl and mix until well combined.
3. Make five equal shapes of patties from mixture and place on a prepared plate.
4. Place plate in the refrigerator for 30 minutes.
5. Spray a large pan with cooking spray and heat over medium heat.
6. Once the pan is hot then add patties

29) Tuna Focaccia

Serves: 8

Cooking Time: 35 minutes

Nutrition: Calories per serving: 185 Fat 14 g Carbs 2.6 g Sugar 0.7 g Protein 13 g Cholesterol 75 mg

Lean Recipe

Ingredients:
- 2 eggs, lightly beaten
- 1 can tuna, flaked
- 1 tsp cayenne pepper
- 1/4 cup mayonnaise
- 1 celery stalk, chopped
- 1 1/2 cups cheddar cheese, shredded
- 1/4 cup sour cream
- Pepper
- Salt

Directions:
1. Preheat the oven to 350 F. Grease muffin tin and set aside.
2. Add all ingredients into the large bowl and mix until well combined and pour into the prepared muffin tin.
3. Bake for 25 minutes.
4. Serve and enjoy.

30) Delicious Tomato Broth

Serves: 2

Cooking Time: 15 minutes

Nutrition: Calories total: 460 Fat 35 g Carbs 13 g Sugar 6 g Protein 24 g Cholesterol 117 mg

Leanest Recipe

Ingredients:
- 14 oz can fire-roasted tomatoes
- 1/2 tsp dried basil
- 1/2 cup heavy cream
- 1/2 cup parmesan cheese, grated
- 1 cup cheddar cheese, grated
- 1 1/2 cups vegetable stock
- 1/4 cup zucchini, grated
- 1/2 tsp dried oregano
- Pepper
- Salt

Directions:
1. Add tomatoes, stock, zucchini, oregano, basil, pepper, and salt into the instant pot and stir well.
2. Seal pot and cook on high pressure for 5 minutes.
3. Release pressure using quick release. Remove lid.
4. Set pot on sauté mode. Add heavy cream, parmesan cheese, and cheddar cheese and stir well and cook until
5. cheese is melted.
6. Serve and enjoy.

31) Baked Salmon Souffle

Serves: 4

Cooking Time: 30 minutes

Nutrition Information: Calories per serving: 216 Fat 11.8 g Carbs 3 g Sugar 0.5 g Protein 24.3 g

Lean Recipe

Ingredients:
- 2 eggs, lightly beaten
- 14 oz can salmon, drained and flaked with a fork
- 1 tbsp garlic, minced
- 1/4 cup almond flour
- 1/2 cup fresh parsley, chopped
- 1 tsp Dijon mustard
- 1/4 tsp pepper
- 1/2 tsp kosher salt

Directions:
1. Preheat the oven to 400 F. Line a baking sheet with parchment paper and set aside.
2. Add all ingredients into the bowl and mix until well combined.
3. Make small patties from mixture and place on a prepared baking sheet.
4. Bake patties for 10 minutes
5. Turn patties and bake for 10 minutes more.
6. Serve and enjoy.

32) Spinach and Tomato Omelette

Serves: 8

Cooking Time: 30 minutes

Nutrition: Calories per serving: 116 Fat 7 g Carbs 1 g Sugar 1 g Protein 10 g

Leanest Recipe

Ingredients:
- 12 eggs
- 2 cups baby spinach, shredded
- 1/4 cup sun-dried tomatoes, sliced
- 1/2 tsp dried basil
- 1/4 cup parmesan cheese, grated
- Pepper
- Salt

Directions:
1. Preheat the oven to 425 F. Grease oven-safe pan and set aside.
2. In a large bowl, whisk eggs with pepper and salt. Add remaining ingredients and stir to combine.
3. Pour egg mixture into the prepared pan and bake for 20 minutes.
4. Slice and serve.

33) Vegan Turkey

Serves: 4

Cooking Time: 15 min

Nutrition: Calories per serving: 194kcal | Fat: 4.3g | Carbohydrates: 0g | Fiber: 0g | Sugar: 0g | Protein: 36.1g

Leanest Recipe

Ingredients:
- Roasted garlic oil (or use any other oil and fresh garlic, chopped) - 4 teaspoons
- Scallion greens (thinly sliced) - 1 cup
- Lean ground turkey - 1 3/4 pound
- Scampi seasoning (or use garlic, lemon, parsley, pepper, onion, salt, and pepper) - 1 tablespoon
- Mixed green lettuce - 8 cup
- To garnish, use lemon wedges from 1 lemon

Directions:
1. Heat the oil over medium-high heat with your pan.
2. Add 3/4 cup of the scallions and cook for a minute.
3. Add the turkey and seasoning.
4. Cook for about 12 min, or until the turkey is fully cooked. Stir and break lumps into smaller pieces while cooking.
5. Add the greens to the serving plates.
6. Add the turkey on top and garnish with the lemon wedges and remaining scallions.

34) *Fettuccine with Turkey Ragù*

Serves: 4

Cooking Time: 20 min

Nutrition: Calories per serving: 179kcal | Fat: 8.5g | Carbohydrates: 8.5g | Fiber: 2.2g | Sugar: 2.2g | Protein: 19.3g

Leaner Recipe

Ingredients:
- Zucchini (spiraled) - 4 cup
- Lean turkey sausage - 1 1/2 pounds (24 oz)
- Tuscan seasoning - 1 tablespoons
- Tomato sauce (no added sugar) - 2 cup
- Fresh parmesan cheese (grated) - 8 tablespoon

Directions:
1. Cut the turkey sausage into 1/2-inch chunks.
2. Place the chunks in a pan and cook over medium-high heat for about 12 min, or until it turns brown. Stir occasionally.
3. Add the Tuscan seasoning and tomato sauce to the pan. Stir thoroughly to coat completely.
4. Increase heat to high and bring mixture to a boil, about 5 min.
5. Add the noodles and toss well.
6. Cook for extra 2 min, or until the noodles become soft and the turkey fully cooked.
7. Transfer to your serving plates and sprinkle over with the parmesan cheese.
8. Serve.

35) *Smoked Range Chicken*

Serves: 6

Cooking Time: 480 min

Nutrition Information:

Calories per serving: 194kcal | Fat: 4.3g | Carbohydrates: 0g | Fiber: 0g | Sugar: 0g | Protein: 36.1g

Leaner Recipe

Ingredients:
- Boneless chicken breasts (skinless) - 2 lbs
- Cinnamon chipotle bbq dust - 2 tablespoon

Directions:
1. Add the chicken to your crock-pot and season.
2. Close with the lid and cook for 8 hours without opening the pot.
3. Open the pot and shred the chicken with 2 forks.
4. Serve.

36) Earl Ground Beef

Serves: 4

Cooking Time: 25 min

Nutrition: Calories per serving: 302kcal | Fat: 11.5g | Carbohydrates: 2.7g | Fiber: 0.6g | Sugar: 1g | Protein: 44.1g

Lean Recipe

Ingredients:
- Lean ground beef - 1 1/2 pounds
- Green bell pepper (diced) - 1/2 cup
- Tomato paste - 2 tablespoons
- Powdered stevia - 1 teaspoon
- Yellow mustard - 1 tablespoon
- Garlic Gusto seasoning - 1 tablespoon
- Cinnamon chipotle seasoning - 1/2 tablespoon
- Red wine vinegar - 1 tablespoon
- Beef broth (low sodium) - 1 cup
- Salt and pepper - to taste

Directions:
1. Add the beef to your pan and cook over medium heat for about 7 min.
2. While cooking, break the beef into smaller pieces.
3. Except the broth, add other ingredients and stir thoroughly to combine well.
4. Then add the broth and increase the heat to medium-high heat.
5. Once it starts boiling, lower the heat to low and simmer for about 15 min with the pot uncovered.
6. Serve.

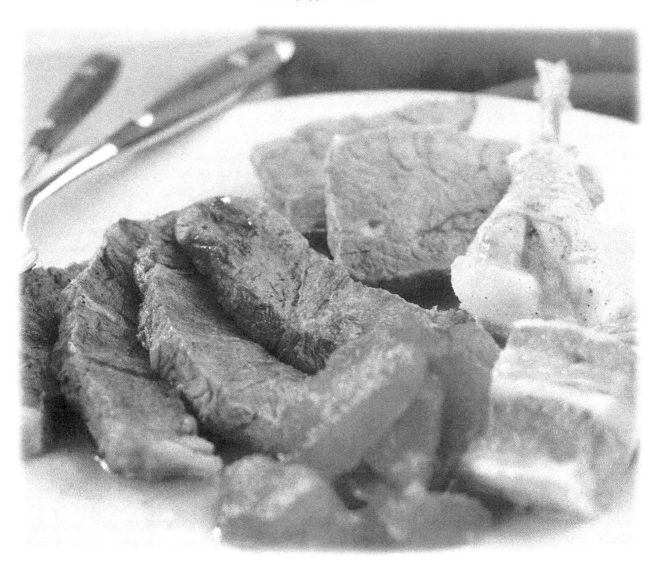

37) A Cup of Cauliflower Taco

Serves: 4

Cooking Time: 15-20 min

Nutrition:

Calories per serving: 275kcal | Fat: 9.9g | Carbohydrates: 6.2g | Fiber: 2.3g | Sugar: 3.6g | Protein: 39g

Lean Recipe

Ingredients:
- Cauliflower (ready-to-cook cauliflower rice) - 1 large head
- Lean ground lamb - 1 1/2 pound
- Low-salt taco seasoning - 1-2 capfuls
- No-sugar, no-flavor added tomatoes (canned, diced) - 2 cup
- Favorite condiments

Directions:
1. Add the ground lamb to a pan and saute for about 12 min over medium-high heat, or until it turns slightly brown.
2. While cooking, break the meat into smaller pieces.
3. Add the seasoning and tomatoes. Stir thoroughly.
4. Lower the heat to low and cook for extra 5 min, or until the liquid reduces by half.
5. Meanwhile, chop the cauliflower to make cauliflower rice.
6. Serve the cauliflower with the lamb mixture, topped with condiments.

38) Prawn Broccoli

Serves: 4

Cooking Time: 10 min

Nutrition Information:

Calories per serving: 340kcal | Fat: 12g | Carbohydrates: 12.4g | Fiber: 3.3g | Sugar: 4.2g | Protein: 45.7g

Leaner Recipe

Ingredients:
- Roasted garlic oil (you can use fresh garlic and any other oil you like) - 4 teaspoons
- Shrimp (wild caught, thawed with shells removed) - 1 3/4 lbs
- Fresh broccoli florets - 2 cup
- Rockin' ranch seasoning - 2 teaspoon
- Garlic and spring onion seasoning - 1 teaspoon
- Chicken broth (low sodium) - 1/3 cup
- Noodles of choice (like hearts of palm noodles) - 4 cup
- Butter - 2 tablespoons

Directions:
1. Add the oil to your pan and heat up over medium-high heat.
2. Add the shrimp and cook each side for about 1 minute.
3. Add the broth and seasonings.
4. Gently stir thoroughly.
5. Add the broccoli and cover pan with the lid.
6. Bring mixture to a boil.
7. Reduce heat to medium and cook for about 2 min extra, or until the broccoli turns bright green.
8. Open the pan and add the butter.
9. Stir and add the noodles.
10. Toss and cook the mixture until it becomes very hot.
11. Then serve hot.

39) Creamy Mushroom Tornado

Serves: 4

Cooking Time: 30 min

Nutrition:

Calories per serving: 341kcal | Fat: 11.6g | Carbohydrates: 4.1g | Fiber: 1.3g | Sugar: 1.6g | Protein: 51.5g

Lean Recipe

Ingredients:
- Sirloin steak (cubed into 1 inch chunks) - 1 1/2 lbs
- Rosemary seasoning - 1 tablespoon (one capful)
- Beef broth (low sodium) - 2 1/2 cup
- Baby portobello mushrooms (sliced) - 4 cup
- Garlic and spring onion seasoning - 1 tablespoon
- Seasoning (or use pepper and salt) - 1 teaspoon
- Guar gum (or other approved thickener) - 1/2 tsp
- Water - 1/4 cup
- Cauliflower mashed potatoes (hot) - 2 cup

Directions:
1. Except the cauliflower mashed potatoes and guar gum, add all ingredients in a pressure cooker and stir thoroughly to combine well.
2. Seal the lid and cook on high for about 15min.
3. Once done, quick release the pressure.
4. Remove the lid and saute.
5. Mix the guar gum and water thoroughly without lumps.
6. Once the mixture in the cooker starts boiling, add the gum mixture and stir.
7. Cook for about 5 min, or until the sauce becomes thick.
8. Season with proper and salt.
9. Serve.

40) Boscaiola Beef Fillet

Serves: 4

Cooking Time: 25 min

Nutrition:

Calories per serving: 214kcal | Fat: 5g | Carbohydrates: 1.2g | Fiber: 0g | Sugar: 0g | Protein: 38.1g

Lean Recipe

Ingredients:
- Seasoning of choice (or a mixture of garlic, parsley, salt, black pepper, and onion) - 1 teaspoons
- Beef tenderloin (you can use chicken breasts or pork tenderloin) - 1 1/2 lbs
- Portobello mushroom caps (chopped into chunks) - 6 cups
- Chicken broth (low sodium) - 1/2 cup
- Garlic Gusto seasoning - 1 tablespoon
- Fresh parsley (for garnish) - optional

Directions:
1. Preheat your oven to 400. Season both sides of the tenderloin.
2. Over high heat, place the oven-safe pan on your stove and grease it with nonstick cooking spray.
3. Once the pan is heated up, place the tenderloins in the pan without touching each other.
4. Cook each side for about 3 min, or until it turns brown. Remove from the pan and set it aside.
5. Leave the pan on the heat and add the broth.
6. Add the mushroom, and garlic seasoning.
7. Scrape the brown bit from the bottom with your wooden spoon.
8. Cook mixture for extra 1 minute. Return the beef to the pan and place in the preheated oven.
9. Cook for about 25 min. Remove from the pan and allow it to cool down a bit for about 3 min.
10. Slice the beef and serve with the sauce and mushroom.

41) Bed of Mushroom with Stir-Fried Tofu

Serves: 2

Cooking Time: 10 min

Nutrition Information:

Calories per serving: 202kcal | Fat: 11g | Carbohydrates: 7g | Fiber: 5g | Sugar: 2g | Protein: 18g

Leanest Recipe

Ingredients:
- Chopped onion - 1/4 cup
- Button mushrooms (chopped) - 1/4 cup
- Extra-firm tofu (chopped) - 8 oz
- Nutritional yeast - 3 teaspoons
- Coconut amino - 1 teaspoon
- Baby spinach - 4 cups
- Grape tomatoes (chopped) - 4–5
- For topping, use sriracha sauce (or another hot sauce) - optional

Directions:
1. Grease your nonstick pan with cooking spray.
2. Add the mushrooms and onion.
3. Saute for about 3 minutes or until the onion becomes translucent.
4. Add the tofu and toss thoroughly to combine well.
5. Cook for extra 2 minutes.
6. Add the coconut amino and yeast.
7. Stir thoroughly to coat completely.
8. Add the tomatoes and spinach and cook until the spinach wilts, about 4 minutes.
9. Top with the sauce and serve.

42) Turkey Sesame Scent

Serves: 4

Cooking Time: 15 min

Nutrition:

Calories per serving: 247kcal | Fat: 9.9g | Carbohydrates: 0.5g | Fiber: 0.3g | Sugar: 0g | Protein: 36.5g

Leanest Recipe

Ingredients:
- Orange oil (or use any other oil and orange zest) - 4 teaspoons
- Turkey meat (skinless and cut into thin slices) - 1 1/2 lbs
- Toasted sesame ginger seasoning - 1 tablespoon

Directions:
1. Sprinkle the seasoning over the turkey.
2. Add the orange oil to a nonstick pan and heat over medium-high heat.
3. Add the turkey and cook each side for about 8 min, or until the turkey is well cooked.
4. Then serve.

43) Lime-Mint Soup

Preparation Time: 5 minutes

Cooking Time: 20 minutes

Servings: 4

Nutrition: Calories: 55; Total fat: 2g; Carbohydrates: 5g; Fiber: 1g; Protein: 5g

Leanest Recipe

Ingredients:
- 4 cups vegetable broth
- ¼ cup fresh mint leaves, roughly chopped
- ¼ cup chopped scallions, white and green parts
- 3 garlic cloves, minced
- 3 tablespoons freshly squeezed lime juice

Directions:
1. In a large stockpot, combine the broth, mint, scallions, garlic, and lime juice. Bring to a boil over medium-high heat.
2. Cover, reduce the heat to low, simmer for 15 minutes, and serve

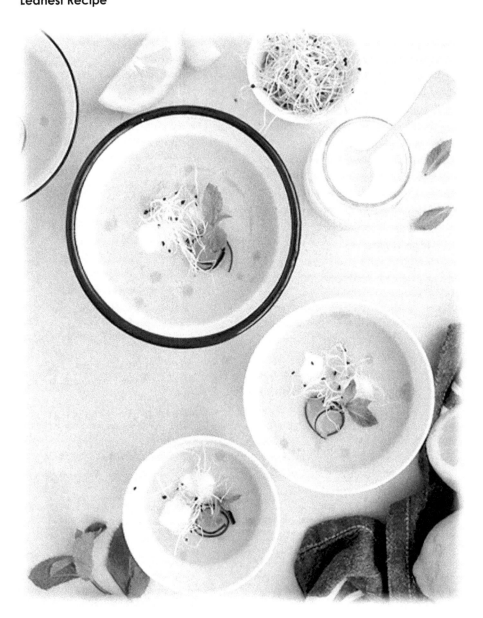

44) Brussels Sprouts Stew

Preparation Time: 10 minutes

Cooking Time: 55 minutes

Servings: 4

Nutrition: Calories: 156 Cal Fat: 3 g Carbs: 22 g Protein: 12 g Fiber: 5.1100 g

Leanest Recipe

Ingredients:
- 35 ounces Brussels sprouts
- 5 medium potatoes, peeled, chopped
- 1 medium onion, peeled, chopped
- 2 carrots, peeled, cubed
- 2 teaspoons smoked paprika
- 1/8 teaspoon ground black pepper
- 1/8 teaspoon salt
- 3 tablespoons caraway seeds
- 1/2 teaspoon red chili powder
- 1 tablespoon nutmeg
- 1 tablespoon olive oil
- 4 ½ cups hot vegetable stock

Directions:
1. Take a large pot, place it over medium-high heat, add oil and when hot, add onion and cook for 1 minute.
2. Then add carrot and potato, cook for 2 minutes, then add Brussel sprouts and cook for 5 minutes.
3. Stir in all the spices, pour in vegetable stock, bring the mixture to boil, switch heat to medium-low and simmer for 45 minutes until cooked and stew reach to desired thickness.
4. Serve straight away.

45) Tomato Pumpkin Soup

Preparation Time: 25 minutes

Cooking Time: 15 minutes

Servings: 4

Nutrition: calories 70; fat 2.7 g; carbohydrates 13.8 g; sugar 6.3 g; protein 1.9 g; cholesterol 0 mg

Leanest Recipe

Ingredients:
- 2 cups pumpkin, diced
- 1/2 cup tomato, chopped
- 1/2 cup onion, chopped
- 1 1/2 tsp curry powder
- 1/2 tsp paprika
- 2 cups vegetable stock
- 1 tsp olive oil
- 1/2 tsp garlic, minced

Directions:
1. In a saucepan, add oil, garlic, and onion and sauté for 3 minutes over medium heat.
2. Add remaining ingredients into the saucepan and bring to boil.
3. Reduce heat and cover and simmer for 10 minutes.
4. Puree the soup using a blender until smooth.
5. Stir well and serve warm.

46) Creamy Squash Soup

Preparation Time: 35 minutes

Cooking Time: 22 minutes

Servings: 8

Nutrition: calories 146; fat 12.6 g; carbohydrates 9.4 g; sugar 2.8 g; protein 1.7 g; cholesterol 0 mg

Leanest Recipe

Ingredients:
- 3 cups butternut squash, chopped
- 1 ½ cups unsweetened coconut milk
- 1 tbsp coconut oil
- 1 tsp dried onion flakes
- 1 tbsp curry powder
- 4 cups water
- 1 garlic clove
- 1 tsp kosher salt

Directions:
1. Add squash, coconut oil, onion flakes, curry powder, water, garlic, and salt into a large saucepan. Bring to boil over high heat.
2. Turn heat to medium and simmer for 20 minutes.
3. Puree the soup using a blender until smooth. Return soup to the saucepan and stir in coconut milk and cook for 2 minutes.
4. Stir well and serve hot.

47) Sautéed Collard greens

Preparation Time: 10 minutes

Cooking Time: 25 minutes

Servings: 4

Nutrition: Calories: 28; Total fat: 1g; Carbohydrates: 4g; Fiber: 2g; Protein: 3g

Leanest Recipe

Ingredients:
- 1½ pounds collard greens
- 1 cup vegetable broth
- ½ teaspoon garlic powder
- ½ teaspoon onion powder
- ⅛ teaspoon freshly ground black pepper

Directions:
1. Remove the hard middle stems from the greens, then roughly chop the leaves into 2-inch pieces.
2. In a large saucepan, mix together the vegetable broth, garlic powder, onion powder, and pepper. Bring to a boil over medium-high heat, then add the chopped greens. Reduce the heat to low, and cover.
3. Cook for 20 minutes, stirring well every 4 to 5 minutes, and serve. (If you notice that the liquid has completely evaporated and the greens are beginning to stick to the bottom of the pan, stir in a few extra tablespoons of vegetable broth or water.)

48) Spinach Soup with Dill and Basil

Preparation Time: 10 minutes

Cooking Time: 25 minutes

Servings: 8

Nutrition: , Carbohydrates 12g Protein 13g Fats 1g Calories

Leanest Recipe

Ingredients:
- 1 pound peeled and diced potatoes
- 1 tablespoon minced garlic
- 1 teaspoon dry mustard
- 6 cups vegetable broth
- 20 ounces chopped frozen spinach
- 2 cups chopped onion
- 1 ½ tablespoons salt
- ½ cup minced dill
- 1 cup basil
- ½ teaspoon ground black pepper

Directions:
1. Whisk onion, garlic, potatoes, broth, mustard, and salt in a pan cook it over medium flame.
2. When it starts boiling, low down the heat and cover it with the lid and cook for 20 minutes.
3. Add the remaining ingredients in it and blend it and cook it for few more minutes and serve it.

49) Cream of Mushroom Soup

Preparation Time: 5 minutes

Cooking Time: 12 minutes

Servings: 6

Nutrition: Calories: 120 Cal Fat: 7 g Carbs: 10 g Protein: 2 g Fiber: 6 g

Leanest Recipe

Ingredients:
- 1 medium white onion, peeled, chopped
- 16 ounces button mushrooms, sliced
- 1 ½ teaspoon minced garlic
- 1/4 cup all-purpose flour
- 1/2 teaspoon ground black pepper
- 1 teaspoon dried thyme
- 1/4 teaspoon nutmeg
- 1/2 teaspoon salt
- 2 tablespoons vegan butter
- 4 cups vegetable broth
- 1 1/2 cups coconut milk, unsweetened

Directions:
1. Take a large pot, place it over medium-high heat, add butter and when it melts, add onions and garlic, stir in garlic and cook for 5 minutes until softened and nicely brown.
2. Then sprinkle flour over vegetables, continue cooking for 1 minute, then add remaining ingredients, stir until mixed and simmer for 5 minutes until thickened.
3. Serve straight away

50) Coconut Watercress Soup

Preparation Time: 10 minutes

Cooking Time: 20 minutes

Servings: 4

Nutrition: calories: 178 protein: 6g; total fat: 10g; carbohydrates: 18g; fiber: 5g

Leanest Recipe

Ingredients:
- teaspoon coconut oil
- 1 onion, diced
- ¾ cup coconut milk

Directions:
1. Preparing the ingredients.
2. Melt the coconut oil in a large pot over medium-high heat. Add the onion and cook until soft, about 5 minutes, then add the peas and the water. Bring to a boil, then lower the heat and add the watercress, mint, salt, and pepper.
3. Cover and simmer for 5 minutes. Stir in the coconut milk, and purée the soup until smooth in a blender or with an immersion blender.
4. Try this soup with any other fresh, leafy green—anything from spinach to collard greens to arugula to Swiss chard.

51) Creamy Celery Soup

Preparation Time: 40 minutes

Cooking Time: 40 minutes

Servings: 4

Nutrition: calories 130; fat 11 g; carbohydrates 9.4 g; sugar 2.5 g; protein 1.6 g; cholesterol 0 mg

Leanest Recipe

Ingredients:
- 6 cups celery
- ½ tsp dill
- 2 cups water
- 1 cup coconut milk
- 1 onion, chopped
- Pinch of salt

Directions:
1. Add all ingredients into the electric pot and stir well.
2. Cover electric pot with the lid and select soup setting.
3. Release pressure using a quick release method than open the lid.
4. Puree the soup using an immersion blender until smooth and creamy.
5. Stir well and serve warm.

52) Cajun Sweet Potatoes

Preparation Time: 5 minutes

Cooking Time: 30 minutes

Servings: 4

Nutrition: Calories: 219; Fat: 3g; Protein: 4g; Carbohydrates: 46g; Fiber: 7g; Sugar: 9g; Sodium: 125mg

Leanest Recipe

Ingredients:
- 2 pounds' sweet potatoes
- 2 teaspoons extra-virgin olive oil
- ½ teaspoon ground cayenne pepper
- ½ teaspoon smoked paprika
- ½ teaspoon dried oregano
- ½ teaspoon dried thyme
- ½ teaspoon garlic powder
- ¼ teaspoon salt (optional)

Directions:
1. Preheat the oven to 400°F. Line a baking sheet with parchment paper.
2. Wash the potatoes, pat dry, and cut into ¾-inch cubes. Transfer to a large bowl, and pour the olive oil over the potatoes.
3. In a small bowl, combine the cayenne, paprika, oregano, thyme, and garlic powder. Sprinkle the spices over the potatoes and combine until the potatoes are well coated. Spread the potatoes on the prepared baking sheet in a single layer. Season with the salt (if using). Roast for 30 minutes, stirring the potatoes after 15 minutes.
4. Divide the potatoes evenly among 4 single-serving containers. Let cool completely before sealing.

53) Mediterranean Hummus Pizza

Preparation Time: 10 minutes

Cooking Time: 30 minutes

Servings: 2 pizzas

Nutrition: Calories: 500; Total fat: 25g; Carbs: 58g; Fiber: 12g;

Leanest Recipe

Ingredients:
- ½ zucchini, thinly sliced
- ½ red onion, thinly sliced
- 1 cup cherry tomatoes, halved
- 2 to 4 tablespoons pitted and chopped black olives
- Pinch sea salt
- Drizzle olive oil (optional)
- 2 prebaked pizza crusts
- ½ cup Classic Hummus
- 2 to 4 tablespoons Cheesy Sprinkle

Directions:
1. Preheat the oven to 400°F. Place the zucchini, onion, cherry tomatoes, and olives in a large bowl, sprinkle them with the sea salt, and toss them a bit.
2. Drizzle with a bit of olive oil (if using), to seal in the flavor and keep them from drying out in the oven.
3. Lay the two crusts out on a large baking sheet.
4. Spread half the hummus on each crust, and top with the veggie mixture and some Cheesy Sprinkle.
5. Pop the pizzas in the oven for 20 to 30 minutes, or until the veggies are soft.

54) Turnip Chips

Preparation Time: 5 minutes

Cooking Time: 50 minutes

Servings: 2

Nutrition: Calories: 136 Fat: 14g Carb: 30g Phosphorus: 50mg Potassium: 356mg Sodium: 71mg Protein: 7g

Leanest Recipe

Ingredients:
- Turnips – 2, peeled and sliced
- Extra virgin olive oil – 1 Tbsp.
- Onion – 1 chopped
- Minced garlic – 1 clove
- Black pepper – 1 tsp.
- Oregano – 1 tsp.
- Paprika - 1 1 tsp.

Directions:
1. Preheat oven to 375F. Grease a baking tray with olive oil.
2. Add turnip slices in a thin layer.
3. Dust over herbs and spices with an extra drizzle of olive oil.
4. Bake 40 minutes. Turning once.

55) Miso Spaghetti Squash

Preparation Time: 5 minutes

Cooking Time: 40 minutes

Servings: 4

Nutrition: Calories: 117; Fat: 2g; Protein: 3g; Carbohydrates: 25g; Fiber: 0g; Sugar: 0g; Sodium: 218mg

Leanest Recipe

Ingredients:
- 1 (3-pound) spaghetti squash
- 1 tablespoon hot water
- 1 tablespoon unseasoned rice vinegar
- 1 tablespoon white miso

Directions:
1. Preheat the oven to 400°F. Line a rimmed baking sheet with parchment paper.
2. Halve the squash lengthwise and place, cut-side down, on the prepared baking sheet. Bake for 35 to 40 minutes, until tender.
3. Cool until the squash is easy to handle.
4. With a fork, scrape out the flesh, which will be stringy, like spaghetti.
5. Transfer to a large bowl. In a small bowl, combine the hot water, vinegar, and miso with a whisk or fork.
6. Pour over the squash. Gently toss with tongs to coat the squash. Divide the squash evenly among 4 single-serving containers.
7. Let cool before sealing the lids.

56) *Tortilla Chips*

Preparation Time: 15 minutes

Cooking Time: 10 minutes

Servings: 6

Nutrition: Calories: 51 Fat: 1g Carb: 9g Phosphorus: 29mg Potassium: 24mg Sodium: 103 mg Protein: 1g

Leanest Recipe

Ingredients:
- Granulated sugar – 2 tsps.
- Ground cinnamon – ½ tsp.
- Pinch ground nutmeg
- Flour tortillas – 3 (6-inch)
- Cooking spray

Directions:
1. Preheat the oven to 350F.
2. Line a baking sheet with parchment paper.
3. In a small bowl, stir together the sugar, cinnamon, and nutmeg.
4. Lay the tortillas on a clean work surface and spray both sides of each lightly with cooking spray.
5. Sprinkle the cinnamon sugar evenly over both sides of each tortilla.
6. Cut the tortillas into 16 wedges each and place them on the baking sheet.
7. Bake the tortilla wedges, turning once, for about 10 minutes or until crisp.
8. Cool the chips serve.

57) *Navy Beans, Spinach, and Artichoke Spread*

Preparation time: 5 minutes

Cooking time: 0 minutes

Servings: 6

Nutrition: calories: 296 fat: 2.1g carbs: 53.2g protein: 21.1g fiber: 18.9g

Lean Recipe

Ingredients:
- 1 (15-ounce / 425-g) can navy beans, rinsed and drained
- 1 (14-ounce / 397-g) can artichoke hearts packed in water, drained
- 1 (10-ounce / 284-g) package frozen spinach, thawed and drained
- ¼ cup nutritional yeast
- 6 cloves garlic, minced
- Sea salt, to taste (optional)
- Pinch of ground nutmeg

Direction:
1. Combine all the ingredients in a food processor. Pulse to mix until creamy and smooth.
2. Smear on the fillings of the tortillas to serve

58) *Broccoli Salad with Cheese*

Preparation Time: 5 Minutes

Cooking Time: 25 Minutes

Servings: 6

Nutrition: Calories 199 Fat 17.4 g Saturated fat 2.9 g Carbohydrates 7.5 g Fiber 2.8 g Protein 5.2 g

Leanest Recipe

Ingredients:
- Two tablespoons sherry vinegar
- ¼ cup olive oil
- Two teaspoons fresh thyme, chopped
- One teaspoon Dijon mustard
- One teaspoon honey
- Salt to taste
- 8 cups broccoli florets
- Two red onions
- ½ cup Parmesan cheese shaved
- ¼ cup pecans

Directions:
1. Mix the sherry vinegar, olive oil, thyme, mustard, honey, and salt in a bowl.
2. In a serving bowl, blend the broccoli florets and onions.
3. Drizzle the dressing on top.
4. Sprinkle with the pecans and Parmesan cheese before serving.

59) Pea Salad

Preparation Time: 40 Minutes

Cooking Time: 0 Minutes

Servings: 6

Nutrition: Calories 214 Fat 8.6 g Saturated fat 1.5 g Carbohydrates 27.3 g Fiber 8.4 g Protein 8 g

Leaner Recipe

Ingredients:
- 1 cup chickpeas, rinsed and drained
- 1 ½ cups peas, divided
- Salt to taste
- Three tablespoons olive oil
- ½ cup buttermilk
- Pepper to taste
- 8 cups pea greens
- Three carrots shaved
- 1 cup snow peas, trimmed

Directions:
1. Add the chickpeas and half of the peas to your food processor.
2. Season with the salt.
3. Pulse until smooth. Set aside.
4. In a bowl, toss the remaining peas in oil, milk, salt, and pepper.
5. Transfer the mixture to your food processor.
6. Process until pureed.
7. Transfer this mixture to a bowl.
8. Arrange the pea greens on a serving plate.
9. Top with the shaved carrots and snow peas.
10. Stir in the pea and milk dressing.
11. Serve with the reserved chickpea hummus.

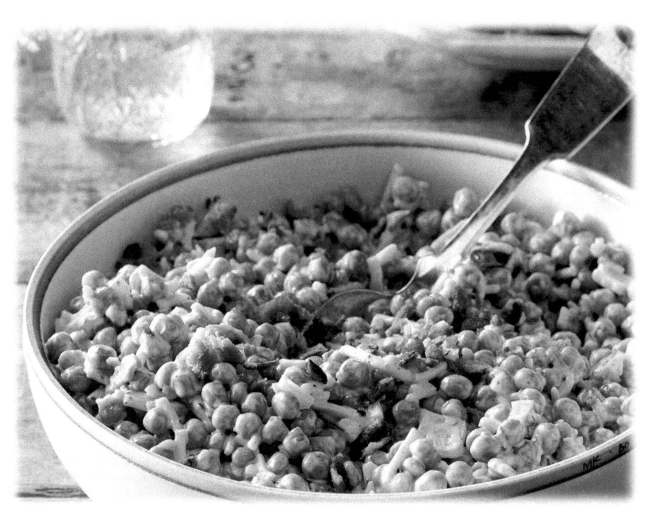

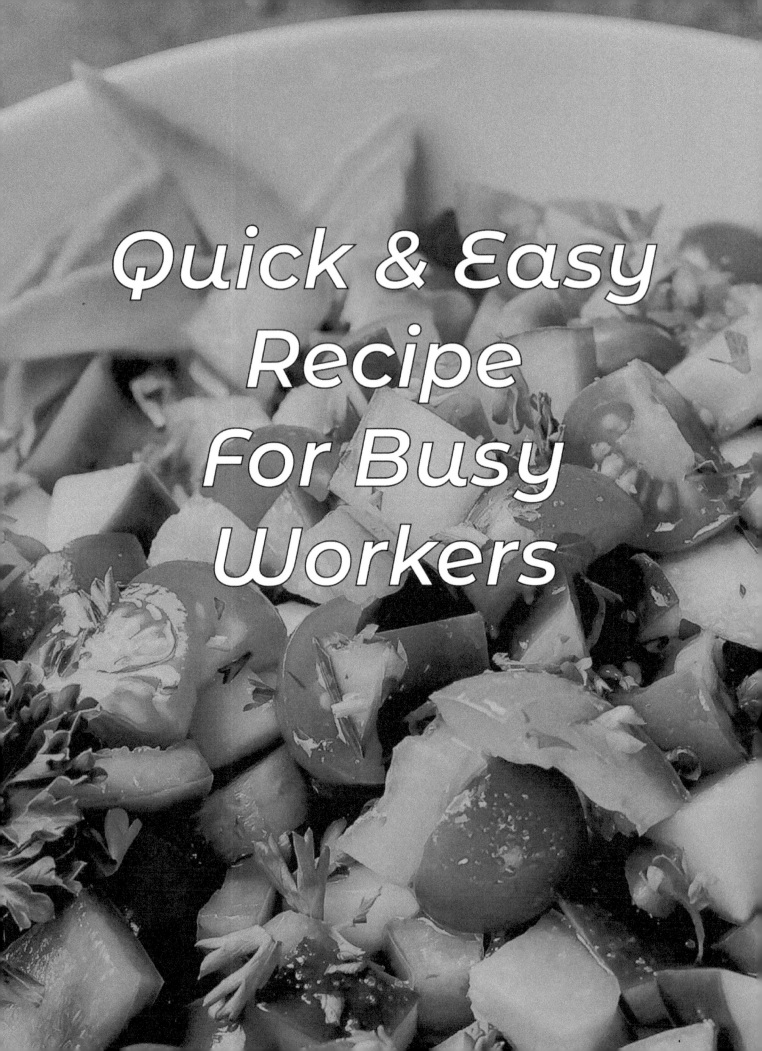

60) Salted Cod Lemon

Serves: 4

Cooking Time: 15 min

Nutrition: Calories total: 250kcal | Fat: 6.2g | Carbohydrates: 0g | Fiber: 0g | Sugar: 0g | Protein: 45.3g

Leanest Recipe

Ingredients:
- Lemon oil - 4 tsp
- Rockin' ranch seasoning (or use a mixture of garlic, onion, lemon, pepper, salt, tarragon, and pepper) - 1 tablespoon
- Cod fillets - 1 3/4 lbs

Directions:
1. Heat the oil over medium-high heat with a pan.
2. Meanwhile, chop the cod into 2-inch chunks.
3. Add the cod to the and cook each side for about 3 minutes or until it becomes flaky and opaque.
4. Serve.

61) Flounder Lemon Sauce

Serves: 4

Cooking Time: 10 min

Nutrition: Calories per serving: 189kcal | Fat: 6.5g | Carbohydrates: 0g | Fiber: 0g | Sugar: 0g | Protein: 30.7g

Leanest Recipe

Ingredients:
- Flounder filets - 1 3/4 pounds
- Lemon oil (or use another oil and lemon zest) - 4 teaspoons
- Citrus dill seasoning (or use any other seasoning you like) - 1-2 tablespoons

Directions:
1. Heat the oil over medium-high heat with a nonstick pan.
2. Add the fish fillets and sprinkle over with the seasoning.
3. Cook each side of the fillets for about 2 min, or until it becomes opaque and flaky.
4. Serve.

62) Scallop Sauce With Butter and Garlic

Serves: 4

Cooking Time: 15 min

Nutrition: Calories per serving: 276kcal | Fat: 13g | Carbohydrates: 4.7g | Fiber: 0g | Sugar: 0g | Protein: 33.4g

Leanest Recipe

Ingredients:
- Dry sea scallops - 2 pounds
- Butter (divided) - 4 tablespoon
- Chicken broth (low sodium) - 3/4 cup
- Garlic & spring onion seasoning - 1 tablespoon
- Fresh lemon juice - 3 tablespoon
- Seasoning (or salt and pepper) - pinch
- To garnish, use mint, fresh parsley, and lemon zest

Directions:
1. Add 1 tablespoon of butter to your pan and heat over high heat.
2. Meanwhile, pat dry the scallops.
3. Add the scallops to the pan when the butter melts.
4. Cook each side for about 3 min, or until it turns brown.
5. Remove from heat and set it aside.
6. Lower the heat to medium and add the juice, broth, and garlic seasoning.
7. Scrape all brown bits at the bottom of the pan.
8. Once the sauce reduces by 1/3, add the remaining butter, and pinch of salt and pepper
9. Whisk mixture together.
10. Return the scallops back to the pan and heat the mixture.
11. Sprinkle over with the parsley, lemon zest, and/or mint.
12. Serve.

63) Baltic Tacos

Serves: 4

Cooking Time: 15 min

Nutrition: Calories per serving: 151kcal | Fat: 1.3g | Carbohydrates: 0.2g | Fiber: 0.1g | Sugar: 0g | Protein: 32.5g

Leanest Recipe

Ingredients:
- Cod (or haddock, wild caught) - 1 3/4 lbs
- Taco seasoning (low sodium) - 1 tablespoon
- Roasted garlic oil - 4 teaspoons
- Preferred taco condiment

Directions:
1. Pat dry the fish and cut it into 1-inch chunks.
2. Sprinkle over with the seasoning and gently toss thoroughly to coat completely.
3. Add the oil over a nonstick pan and heat over medium-high heat.
4. Add the fish and cook for additional 12 min, or until the fish breaks apart into flakes and turns opaque.
5. Then serve with the condiments.

64) Garlic Green Beans Sautéed with Parmesan

Serves: 4

Cooking Time: 10 min

Nutrition: Calories per serving: 84kcal | Fat: 5g | Carbohydrates: 7.8g | Fiber: 3.7g | Sugar: 1.5g | Protein: 4g

Leanest recipe

Ingredients:
- Green beans (with ends trimmed) - 1 1/2 pounds
- Garlic and spring onion seasoning - 1/2 tablespoon
- Roasted garlic oil (or any other oil you like) - 1 tablespoon
- Parmesan cheese (freshly grated) - 4 tablespoons

Directions:
1. Add the green beans to a pot.
2. Add up to 1 inch of water to the pot.
3. Sprinkle over with the seasoning.
4. Cover the pot and place it on your stove.
5. Cook over high heat and bring to boil, about 7 min, or until the beans steams and becomes crisp tender.
6. Drain the water and drizzle over with the garlic oil and pepper and salt.
7. Sprinkle over with the Parmesan cheese.
8. Serve.

65) Paprika Pork in Garlic Sauce

Serves: 4

Cooking Time: 15 min

Nutrition: Calories per serving: 239kcal | Fat: 8.1g | Carbohydrates: 7.7g | Fiber: 0.8g | Sugar: 6.8g | Protein: 32.2g

Leaner Recipe

Ingredients:
- Boneless pork loin (skinless) - 18 ounces
- Ground paprika - 4 teaspoons
- Seasoning (or use salt, garlic, pepper, and onion) - 1 tablespoon
- Roasted garlic oil - 1/2 - 1 tablespoon
- Plain Greek yogurt (unflavored) - 12 ounces
- Garlic and spring onion seasoning - 1/2 - 1 tablespoon
- Cauliflower rice (steamed) - 4 cups (optional)

Directions:
1. Cut the meat into 1-inch chunks.
2. Place the meat in a bowl and sprinkle over with the seasoning. Toss thoroughly to coat.
3. Add the garlic oil to a pan and heat over medium-high heat.
4. Add the pork to the heated pan and cook for about 7 min, or until it turns brown. Remember to stir occasionally.
5. Add the Garlic and Spring Onion and yogurt to the pan.
6. Lower the heat to medium and simmer for about 5 min, or until the sauce becomes thick. Stir often.
7. Serve over the cauliflower rice.

66) *Chicken Stuffed with Cauliflower*

Serves: 4

Cooking Time: 25 min

Nutrition: Calories per serving: 258kcal | Fat: 6.4g | Carbohydrates: 13.9g | Fiber: 3.5g | Sugar: 5.4g | Protein: 36g

Leaner Recipe

Ingredients:
- Skinless and boneless chicken breasts (1-inch chunks) - 2 pounds
- Seasoning (or use salt & pepper) - 1 teaspoon
- Roasted garlic oil (or any oil with fresh garlic) - 4 teaspoon
- Diced tomatoes (no added sugar) - 3 cup
- Cajun seasoning (or use any blackening seasoning) - 2 teaspoons
- Fresh lime juice - 2 tablespoon
- Cooked cauliflower rice - 3 cup
- To garnish, use sliced scallion greens and fresh cilantro

Directions:
1. Pat dry the chicken with paper towel and season with pepper and salt.
2. Add the oil to a pan and heat over medium-high heat.
3. Add the chicken to the pan and cook on each side for about 7 min, or until they turn brown.
4. Remove the chicken breasts and set them aside.
5. Add the seasonings and tomatoes to the pan.
6. Bring mixture to a boil and scrape all the brown bits from the bottom of the pan.
7. Once it starts to boil, lower heat to medium and simmer for about 10 min.
8. Return the chicken breasts to the pan and cook for extra 15 min, or until it is fully cooked.
9. Serve.

67) *Spicy Mushroom Collard Wraps*

Servings: 4

Cooking Time: 16 minutes

Nutrition: Calories:380, Total Fat:34.8g, Saturated Fat:19.9g, Total Carbs:10g, Dietary Fiber:5g, Sugar:5g, Protein:10g, Sodium:395mg

Leanest Recipe

Ingredients:
- 2 tbsp avocado oil
- 1 large yellow onion, chopped
- 2 garlic cloves, minced
- Salt and ground black pepper to taste
- 1 small jalapeño pepper, deseeded and finely chopped
- 1 ½ lb mushrooms, cut into 1-inch cubes
- 1 cup cauliflower rice
- 2 tsp hot sauce
- 8 collard leaves
- ¼ cup plain unsweetened yogurt for topping

Directions:
1. Heat 2 tablespoons of avocado oil in a large deep skillet; add and sauté the onion until softened, 3 minutes.
2. Pour in the garlic, salt, black pepper, and jalapeño pepper; Cooking Time: until fragrant, 1 minute.
3. Mix in the mushrooms and Cooking Time: both sides, 10 minutes.
4. Add the cauliflower rice, and hot sauce. Sauté until the cauliflower slightly softens, 2 to 3 minutes. Adjust the taste with salt and black pepper.
5. Lay out the collards on a clean flat surface and spoon the curried mixture onto the middle part of the leaves, about 3 tablespoons per leaf. Spoon the plain yogurt on top, wrap the leaves, and serve immediately.

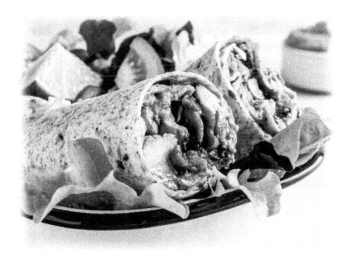

68) *Tofu Scalloppini & Lemon*

Servings: 4

Cooking Time: 21 minutes

Nutrition: Calories:214, Total Fat:15.6g, Saturated Fat:2.5g, Total Carbs:12g, Dietary Fiber:2g, Sugar:6g, Protein:9g, Sodium:280mg

Leanest Recipe

Ingredients:
- 1½ lb thin cut tofu chops, boneless
- Salt and ground black pepper to taste
- 1 tbsp avocado oil
- 3 tbsp butter
- 2 tbsp capers
- 1 cup vegetable broth
- ½ lemon, juiced + 1 lemon, sliced
- 2 tbsp freshly chopped parsley

Directions:
1. Heat the avocado oil in a large skillet over medium heat. Season the tofu chops with salt and black pepper; Cooking Time: in the oil on both sides until brown and cooked through, 12 to 15 minutes. Transfer to a plate, cover with another plate, and keep warm.
2. Add the butter to the pan to melt and Cooking Time: the capers until hot and sizzling stirring frequently to avoid burning, 3 minutes.
3.
4. Pour in the vegetable broth and lemon juice, use a spatula to scrape any bits stuck to the bottom of the pan, and allow boiling until the sauce reduces by half.
5. Add the tofu back to the sauce, arrange the lemon slices on top, and sprinkle with half of the parsley. Allow simmering for 3 minutes.
6. Plate the food, garnish with the remaining parsley, and serve warm with creamy mashed cauliflower.

69) *Creamy Fettuccine with Peas*

Serving: 4

Cooking Time: 10 minutes

Nutrition: Calories 654 Fats 23.7g | Carbs 101.9g Protein 18.2g

Lean Recipe

Ingredients:
- 16 oz whole-wheat fettuccine
- Salt and black pepper to taste
- ¾ cup flax milk
- ½ cup cashew butter, room temperature
- 1 tbsp olive oil
- 2 garlic cloves, minced
- 1 ½ cups frozen peas
- ½ cup chopped fresh basil

Directions:
1. Add the fettuccine and 10 cups of water to a large pot, and Cooking Time: over medium heat until al dente, 10 minutes.
2. Drain the pasta through a colander and set aside. In a bowl, whisk the flax milk, cashew butter, and salt until smooth. Set aside.
3. Heat the olive oil in a large skillet and sauté the garlic until fragrant, 30 seconds.
4. Mix in the peas, fettuccine, and basil. Toss well until the pasta is well-coated in the sauce and season with some black pepper.
5. Dish the food and serve warm.

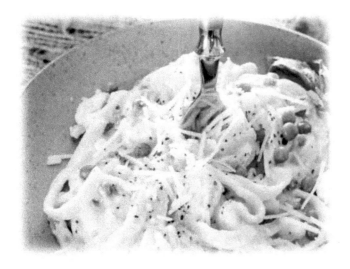

70) Broccoli Salad with Cheese

Servings: 6

Cooking Time: 25 Minutes

Nutrition: Calories 199 Fat 17.4 g Saturated fat 2.9 g Carbohydrates 7.5 g Fiber 2.8 g Protein 5.2 g

Leaner Recipe

Ingredients:
- Two tablespoons sherry vinegar
- ¼ cup olive oil
- Two teaspoons fresh thyme, chopped
- One teaspoon Dijon mustard
- One teaspoon honey
- Salt to taste
- 8 cups broccoli florets
- Two red onions
- ½ cup Parmesan cheese shaved
- ¼ cup pecans

Directions:
1. Mix the sherry vinegar, olive oil, thyme, mustard, honey, and salt in a bowl.
2. In a serving bowl, blend the broccoli florets and onions.
3. Drizzle the dressing on top.
4. Sprinkle with the pecans and Parmesan cheese before serving.

71) Creamy Cauliflower Chipotle Spread

Servings: 6

Cooking time: 5 minutes

Nutrition: calories: 235 fat: 1.8g carbs: 39.7g protein: 8.8g fiber: 8.2g

Leanest Recipe

Ingredients:
- 1½ cups cauliflower florets
- 2 chipotle peppers in adobo sauce
- ½ cup low-sodium vegetable soup
- Sea salt and black pepper, to taste (optional)
- 3 shallots, minced
- 2 cloves garlic, minced
- ¼ cup dry white wine

Direction:
1. Cook the cauliflower in a steamer for 10 minutes or until soft. Transfer the cauliflower in a food processor. Add the chipotle peppers, then pour in the vegetable soup and sprinkle with salt (if desired). Pulse to purée until creamy and smooth. Set aside.
2. Add the shallots in a skillet and sauté over medium heat for 5 minutes or until translucent.
3. Add the garlic and sauté for 1 more minute or until fragrant.
4. Pour the wine in the skillet and cook until the liquid is almost absorbed.
5. Reduce the heat to medium-low and pour in the puréed cauliflower and chipotle peppers. Cover and simmer for 5 minutes until it becomes thick. Stir occasionally.
6. Smear on the fillings of the tortillas or pitas to serve.

72) Red Potatoes and Green Beans

Servings: 2

Cooking Time: 15 minutes

Nutrition: Calories 242 Total Fat 7.6 g Saturated 2.6 g Cholesterol 0 mg Sodium 115 mg Total Carbs 29.1 g Fiber 4.6 g Sugar 6 g Protein 14.2 g

Leaner Recipe

Ingredients
- 1 pound red potatoes, cut into wedges
- 1 pound green beans
- 2 garlic cloves, minced
- 2 tablespoons olive oil
- Salt and black pepper to the taste
- ½ teaspoon oregano, dried

Directions:
1. In a pan that fits your Air Fryer, combine potatoes with green beans, garlic, oil, salt, pepper and oregano, toss, introduce in your Air Fryer and cook at 380° F for 15 minutes.
2. Divide between plates and serve as a side dish.

73) Green Beans Side Salad

Servings: 2

Cooking Time: 15 minutes

Nutrition: Calories 242 Total Fat 7.6 g Saturated 2.6 g Cholesterol 0 mg Sodium 115 mg Total Carbs 29.1 g Fiber 4.6 g Sugar 6 g Protein 14.2 g

Leaner Recipe

Ingredients
- 1-pint cherry tomatoes
- 1 pound green beans
- 2 tablespoons olive oil
- Salt and black pepper to the taste

Directions:
1. In a bowl, mix cherry tomatoes with green beans, olive oil, salt and pepper, toss, and transfer to a pan that fits your Air Fryer and cook at 400 °F for 15 minutes.
2. Divide between plates and serve as a side dish.

74) Corn Bread

Preparation Time: 10 minutes

Cooking Time: 20 minutes

Servings: 10

Nutrition: Calories: 198 Fat: 5g Carb: 34g Phosphorus: 88mg Potassium: 94mg Sodium: 25mg Protein: 4g

Leaner Recipe

Ingredients:
- Cooking spray for greasing the baking dish
- Yellow cornmeal – 1 ¼ cups
- All-purpose flour – ¾ cup
- Baking soda substitute – 1 tbsp.
- Granulated sugar – ½ cup
- Eggs – 2
- Unsweetened, unfortified rice milk – 1 cup
- Olive oil – 2 Tbsps.

Directions:
1. Preheat the oven to 425F.
2. Lightly spray an 8-by-8-inch baking dish with cooking spray. Set aside.
3. In a medium bowl, stir together the cornmeal, flour, baking soda substitute, and sugar.
4. In a small bowl, whisk together the eggs, rice milk, and olive oil until blended.
5. Add the wet ingredients to the dry ingredients and stir until well combined.
6. Pour the batter into the baking dish and bake for 20 minutes or until golden and cooked through.
7. Serve warm.

75) Smoky Coleslaw

Preparation Time: 10 minutes

Cooking Time: 0 minute

Servings: 6

Nutrition: Calories: 73; Fat: 4g; Protein: 1g; Carbohydrates: 8g; Fiber: 2g; Sugar: 5g; Sodium: 283mg

Leanest Recipe

Ingredients:
- 1 pound shredded cabbage
- ⅓ cup vegan mayonnaise
- ¼ cup unseasoned rice vinegar
- 3 tablespoons plain vegan yogurt or plain soymilk
- 1 tablespoon vegan sugar
- ½ teaspoon salt
- ¼ teaspoon freshly ground black pepper
- ¼ teaspoon smoked paprika
- ¼ teaspoon chipotle powder

Directions:
1. Put the shredded cabbage in a large bowl. In a medium bowl, whisk the mayonnaise, vinegar, yogurt, sugar, salt, pepper, paprika, and chipotle powder.
2. Pour over the cabbage, and mix with a spoon or spatula and until the cabbage shreds are coated. Divide the coleslaw evenly among 6 single-serving containers. Seal the lids.

76) *Vegan Chocolate Orange Truffles*

Preparation Time: 15 minutes

Cooking Time: 0 minute

Servings: 16

Nutrition: 58 calories, 1g proteins, 2g fats, 11g carbs

Leanest Recipe

Ingredients:
- ½ lb pitted dates
- 2 ounces' almond meal
- 2 tablespoons unsweetened cocoa powder
- 2 teaspoons cocoa powder (for rolling the balls)
- 2 tablespoons orange juice
- 1 lemon peel

Directions:
1. Place pitted dates, almond meal, cocoa powder, orange juice, and lemon zest in a food processor or a powerful blender. Mix well.
2. Make the mixture into balls using your hands. Make 16 truffles

77) *Broccoli Salad*

Preparation Time: 5 minutes

Cooking Time: 25 minutes

Servings: 6

Nutrition: Calories 199 Fat 17.4 g Saturated fat 2.9 g Carbohydrates 7.5 g Fiber 2.8 g Protein 5.2 g

Leanest Recipe

Ingredients:
- 2 tablespoons sherry vinegar
- ¼ cup olive oil
- 2 teaspoons fresh thyme, chopped
- 1 teaspoon Dijon mustard
- 1 teaspoon honey
- Salt to taste
- 8 cups broccoli florets, steamed or roasted
- 2 red onions, sliced thinly
- ½ cup Parmesan cheese, shaved
- ¼ cup pecans, toasted and chopped

Directions:
1. Mix the sherry vinegar, olive oil, thyme, mustard, honey and salt in a bowl.
2. In a serving bowl, combine the broccoli florets and onions.
3. Drizzle the dressing on top.
4. Sprinkle with the pecans and Parmesan cheese before serving.

78) *Zucchini Pasta Salad*

Preparation Time: 4 minutes

Cooking Time: 0 minute

Servings: 15

Nutrition: Calories 299 Fat 24.7 g Saturated fat 5.1 g Carbohydrates 11.6 g Fiber 2.8 g Protein 7 g

Leanest Recipe

Ingredients:
- 5 tablespoons olive oil
- 2 teaspoons Dijon mustard
- 3 tablespoons red-wine vinegar
- 1 clove garlic, grated
- 2 tablespoons fresh oregano, chopped
- 1 shallot, chopped
- ¼ teaspoon red pepper flakes
- 16 oz. zucchini noodles
- ¼ cup Kalamata olives, pitted
- 3 cups cherry tomatoes, sliced in half
- ¾ cup Parmesan cheese, shaved

Directions:
1. Mix the olive oil, Dijon mustard, red-wine vinegar, garlic, oregano, shallot and red pepper flakes in a bowl.
2. Stir in the zucchini noodles.
3. Sprinkle on top the olives, tomatoes and Parmesan cheese.

79) *Polenta with Pears and Cranberries*

Preparation Time: 5 minutes

Cooking Time: 10 minutes

Servings: 4 bowls

Nutrition: Calories: 200 Fat: 13 g Protein: 4 g Carbs: 17 g Fiber: 3g

Leanest Recipe

Ingredients:
- 2 pears, cored, diced
- 1 tsp ground cinnamon
- ¼ cup brown rice syrup
- 1 cup dried or fresh cranberries
- 1 batch basic polenta

Directions:
1. In a medium saucepan, heat the brown rice syrup and add the cranberries, cinnamon, and pears. Cook. Stir continuously until the pears are tender. This should take about 10 minutes.
2. Divide the polenta in 4 individual bowls. Top with the pear compote and serve.
3. Enjoy!

Fuelings Recipe

80) Light Chocolate Bars

Serves: 16

Cooking Time: 20 minutes

Nutrition: Calories per serving: 230 Fat 24 g Carbs 7.5 g Sugar 0.1 g Protein 6 g Cholesterol 29 mg

Ingredients:
- 15 oz cream cheese, softened
- 15 oz unsweetened dark chocolate
- 1 tsp vanilla
- 10 drops liquid stevia

Directions:
1. Grease 8-inch square dish and set aside.
2. Melt chocolate in a saucepan over low heat. Add stevia and vanilla and stir well.
3. Remove pan from heat and set aside.
4. Add cream cheese into the blender and blend until smooth.
5. Add melted chocolate mixture into the cream cheese and blend until just combined.
6. Transfer mixture into the prepared dish and spread evenly and place in the refrigerator until firm. Slice and serve.

81) Mexican Pudding

Serves: 2

Cooking Time: 20 minutes

Nutrition: Calories total: 360 Fat 33 g Carbs 13 g Sugar 5 g Protein 6 g Cholesterol 0 mg

Ingredients:
- 4 tbsp chia seeds
- 1 cup unsweetened coconut milk
- 1/2 cup raspberries

Directions:
1. Add raspberry and coconut milk into a blender and blend until smooth.
2. Pour mixture into the glass jar.
3. Add chia seeds in a jar and stir well.
4. Seal the jar with a lid and shake well and place in the refrigerator for 3 hours.
5. Serve chilled and enjoy.

82) Brazilian Pudding

Serves: 8

Cooking Time: 20 minutes

Nutrition: Calories total: 317 Fat 30 g Carbs 9 g Sugar 0.5 g Protein 3 g Cholesterol 0 mg

Ingredients:
- 2 ripe avocados, peeled, pitted and cut into pieces
- 1 tbsp fresh lime juice
- 14 oz can coconut milk
- 2 tsp liquid stevia
- 2 tsp vanilla

Directions:
1. Add all ingredients into the blender and blend until smooth.
2. Serve immediately and enjoy.

83) Peanut Butter Delight

Serves: 8

Cooking Time: 10 minutes

Nutrition: Calories total: 101 Fat 5 g Carbs 14 g Sugar 7 g Protein 3 g Cholesterol 0 mg

Ingredients:
- 1/4 cup peanut butter
- 4 overripe bananas, chopped
- 1/3 cup cocoa powder
- 1/4 tsp vanilla extract
- 1/8 tsp salt

Directions:
1. Add all ingredients into the blender and blend until smooth.
2. Serve immediately and enjoy.

84) Raspberry Ice Cream

Serves: 2

Cooking Time: 10 minutes

Nutrition: Calories total: 144 Fat 11 g Carbs 10 g Sugar 4 g Protein 2 g Cholesterol 41 mg

Ingredients:
- 1 cup frozen raspberries
- 1/2 cup heavy cream
- 1/8 tsp stevia powder

Directions:
1. Add all ingredients into the blender and blend until smooth.
2. Serve immediately and enjoy.

85) Chocolate Almond Bites

Serves: 4

Cooking Time: 26 minutes

Nutrition: Calories per serving: 82 Fat 2 g Carbs 11 g Sugar 5 g Protein 7 g Cholesterol 16 mg

Ingredients:
- 1 cup bananas, overripe
- 1/2 cup almond butter, melted
- 1 scoop protein powder
- 2 tbsp unsweetened cocoa powder

Directions:
1. Preheat the air fryer to 325 F. Grease air fryer baking pan and set aside.
2. Add all ingredients into the blender and blend until smooth.
3. Pour batter into the prepared pan and place in the air fryer basket and cook for 16 minutes.
4. Serve and enjoy.

86) Butter Creamy Fudge

Serves: 18

Cooking Time: 10 minutes

Nutrition: Calories total: 197 Fat 16 g Carbs 7 g Sugar 1 g Protein 4 g Cholesterol 0 mg

Ingredients:
- 3/4 cup creamy almond butter
- 1 1/2 cups unsweetened chocolate chips

Directions:
1. Line 8*4-inch pan with parchment paper and set aside.
2. Add chocolate chips and almond butter into the double boiler and cook over medium heat until the chocolate-
3. butter mixture is melted. Stir well.
4. Pour mixture into the prepared pan and place in the freezer until set.
5. Slice and serve.

87) Cocoa Chocolate Mousse

Serves: 4

Cooking Time: 10 minutes

Nutrition: Calories total: 254 Fat 25 g Carbs 7 g Sugar 0.4 g Protein 5 g Cholesterol 83 mg

Ingredients:
- 1/2 cup unsweetened cocoa powder
- 1 1/4 cup heavy cream
- 5 drop stevia
- 4 oz cream cheese
- 1/2 tsp vanilla

Directions:
1. Add all ingredients to the blender and blend until smooth and.
2. Pipe mixture into the serving glasses and place them in the refrigerator for 1 hour.
3. Serve chilled and enjoy.

88) Almond Bites

Serves: 7

Cooking Time: 28 minutes

Nutrition: Calories per serving: 88 Fat 7 g Carbs 3 g Sugar 1 g Protein 3 g Cholesterol 0 mg

Ingredients:
- 6 oz almond butter
- 1/3 cup pumpkin puree
- 1/4 tsp pumpkin pie spice
- 1 tsp liquid stevia

Directions:
1. Preheat the oven to 350 F. Line baking sheet with parchment paper and set aside.
2. Add all ingredients into the food processor and process until just combined.
3. Drop spoonfuls of mixture onto the prepared baking sheet.
4. Bake for 18 minutes.
5. Let the cookies cool completely.
6. Serve and enjoy.

89) Coffe Blend Mousse

Serves: 8

Cooking Time: 20 minutes

Calories per serving: 211 Fat 22 g Carbs 7 g Sugar 0.2 g Protein 3 g

Ingredients:
- 1/2 cup coffee strong brewed, cooled
- 2 cups heavy whipping cream
- 6 oz unsweetened chocolate, chopped
- 1 tsp coffee extract

Directions:
1. In a large bowl, whip heavy cream and set aside.
2. Melt chocolate in a microwave-safe bowl.
3. Add coffee and coffee extract in melted chocolate and stir well.
4. Pour chocolate mixture into the whipped cream and stir until just combined.
5. Place in refrigerator for 30 minutes.
6. Serve and enjoy.

90) Light Cake

Serves: 10

Cooking Time: 65 minutes

Nutrition: Calories total: 211 Fat 17 g Carbs 8 g Sugar 5 g Protein 3 g Cholesterol 89 mg

Ingredients:
- 4 eggs
- 1/4 cup cream cheese
- 1/4 cup butter
- 1 tsp baking powder
- 1 tbsp coconut flour
- 1 cup almond flour
- 1/2 cup sour cream
- 1 tsp vanilla
- 1 cup monk fruit sweetener

Directions:
1. Preheat the oven to 350 F. Grease 9-inch cake pan and set aside.
2. In a large bowl, mix together almond flour, baking powder, and coconut flour.
3. In a separate bowl, add cream cheese and butter and microwave for 30 seconds. Stir well and microwave for 30
4. seconds more.
5. Stir in sour cream, vanilla, and sweetener. Stir well.
6. Pour cream cheese mixture into the almond flour mixture and stir until just combined.
7. Add eggs in batter one by one and stir until well combined.
8. Pour batter into the prepared cake pan and bake for 55 minutes.
9. Remove cake from the oven and let it cool completely.
10. Slice and serve.

91) Cinnamon Explosion

Serves: 6

Cooking Time: 15 minutes

Nutrition: Calories total: 264; Protein: 6.7g; Carbs: 54.1g; Fat: 2.4g Sugar: 0.3g

Ingredients:
- 1 packet Medifast Cinnamon Pretzels
- 1/4 teaspoon baking powder
- 1 tablespoon eggbeaters or egg substitute
- 1 tablespoon water
- 1/8 teaspoon cinnamon
- 1 packet stevia

Directions:
1. Preheat the oven to 3500F.
2. While still in the bag, break the pretzels into smaller pieces or place them in a food processor and grind them
3. into powder.
4. Transfer to a bowl and add in the baking powder, eggbeaters, and water. Stir until well combined. Add the rest
5. of the ingredients and mix until a dough is formed.
6. Press the dough into a baking dish.
7. Place in the oven and bake for 15 minutes.
8. Remove from the oven and allow to cool before slicing into bars.

92) Greek Breakfast

Serves: 2

Cooking Time: 5 minutes

Nutrition: Calories per serving:198; Protein: 11.1g; Carbs: 31.2g; Fat: 3.1g Sugar: 15.4g

Ingredients:
- 12 ounces plain low-fat Greek yogurt
- 2 packets zero-calorie sugar substitute
- 1 sachet Optavia Essential Red Berry Crunchy O's Cereal

Directions:
1. Line an 8x8 baking dish with non-stick foil. Set aside.
2. In a bowl, combine the Greek yogurt and sugar substitute.
3. Spread the Greek yogurt mixture into the prepared baking dish and sprinkle with the Red Berry Crunchy O's
4. Cereal on top.
5. Put in the freezer for 5 hours until the bark is hard.
6. Break the bark with a sharp knife into smaller pieces.

93) Diet Tomato Cookies

Serves: 2

Cooking Time: 15 minutes

Nutrition: Calories total: 337; Protein: 9.5g; Carbs: 38.5g; Fat: 5.3g Sugar: 4.3g

Ingredients:
- 1 sachet Optavia Buttermilk Cheddar and Herb Biscuit
- 2 tablespoons water
- 1 tablespoon tomato sauce
- 1 tablespoon low fat cheese, shredded

Directions:
1. Preheat the oven or toaster to 3500F for 5 minutes. In a bowl, stir the Optavia Buttermilk Cheddar and Herb Biscuit with water to form a thick paste. Spread into a
2. thin circle on a baking tray lined with parchment paper. Cook for 10 minutes to harden. Once harden, spread tomato sauce on top and cheese. Bake for another 5 minutes.

94) Diet Haystacks

Serves: 3

Cooking Time: 5 minutes

Nutrition: Calories per serving: 157; Protein: 16.3g; Carbs: 46g; Fat: 12.3g Sugar: 3.5g

Ingredients:
- 1 packet Optavia or Medifast Hot Cocoa or Brownie Mix
- 3 tablespoons water
- 1 packet Medifast Cinnamon Pretzel Sticks, crushed
- 2 tablespoons Peanut Butter Powder
- 1 packet Stevia

Directions:
1. In a small bowl, mix together the Medifast Hot Cocoa or Brownie Mix with water to form a paste.
2. Add the rest of the ingredients. Stir until well-combined.
3. Drop a tall pile (about 5 inches) of the mixture into a plate and freeze for at least 30 minutes to an hour or until it hardens.

95) Cheesecake Cookies

Serves: 3

Cooking Time: 2 minutes

Nutrition: Calories per serving: 242; Protein:22.1 g; Carbs: 35.2g; Fat:5.7 g Sugar: 8.2g

Ingredients:
- 1 packet Optavia Brownie Mix
- 5 tablespoons water
- 1 packet Optavia Banana Pudding Mix
- 2 tablespoons light cream cheese

Directions:
1. Combine the Optavia Brownie Mix and 2 tablespoons of water in a bowl until a thick paste is formed.
2. Spread the mixture into a baking dish or plate until thick round circles are formed.
3. Microwave for 1 minute and 30 seconds until the cookie hardens. Set aside to cool completely.
4. In another bowl, combine the remaining ingredients and mix until a smooth batter is formed.
5. Spread the batter on to the cookies.

96) Borough Eggs

Serves: 3

Cooking Time: 5 minutes

Nutrition: Calories per serving: 169; Protein: 5.1g; Carbs: 27g; Fat: 2g Sugar: 13g

Ingredients:
- 1 packet Medifast Hot Cocoa Powder
- 2 tablespoons water
- 1 tablespoon Walden Farms Marshmallow Crème
- 1 tablespoon PB2

Directions:
1. In a bowl, combine the Medifast Hot Cocoa Powder and water. Spoon half of the mixture on a plate and form an oval shape.
2. In another bowl, combine the Marshmallow Crème and PB2. Spoon on top of the oval shaped Cocoa Powder mixture.
3. Pour the remaining half of the chocolate syrup over the top of the Marshmallow Crème mixture.
4. Place in the fridge for at least an hour for the mixture to harden.

97) Tasty Diet Lemon Meringue

Serves: 4

Cooking Time: 2 minutes

Nutrition: Calories per serving: 224; Protein: 11.9g; Carbs: 34.4g; Fat: 11.2g Sugar: 10.1g

Ingredients:
- 2 packets Optavia Essential Lemon Crisp Bars
- 1 1/2 cups low fat plain Greek yogurt
- 1 3-ounce box sugar-free lemon gelatin
- 1/2 teaspoon lime zest

Directions:
1. Line a muffin tin with cupcake liner.
2. Break the Optavia Essential Lemon Crisp Bars into thirds and place in a bowl. Microwave for 15 seconds until
3. soft.
4. Press the softened bars into the cupcake liners to form a crust.
5. In another microwavable-safe bowl, mix the yogurt, gelatin, and lime zest. Microwave for 2 minutes and pour
6. the mixture into the crust-lined cupcake liners.
7. Chill for an hour before serving.

98) Peanut Butter Crunch Bars

Cooking Time: 5 minutes

Servings: 4

Ingredients:
- 1 Optavia chocolate pudding (1 fueling)
- 3 Optavia Peanut Butter Snap Bars (3 fuelings)

Directions:
1. Make pudding in a medium-sized bowl as instructed, and set aside.
2. Place the peanut butter crunch bars into a separate bowl and microwave for around 20 seconds.
3. In the prepared pudding, pour melted crunch bars and stir until mixed.
4. Transfer the mixture onto a cookie sheet lined with parchment paper, and spread uniformly into a rectangular shape for making bars to desired thickness.
5. Four silicone muffin cup holders can also be used, and the mixture split equally between the cups.
6. Freeze for 2 hours minimum.
7. When freezing on a cookie sheet or peeling back silicone cup, break it into four equal portions and enjoy!

99) Grilled Cheese Tomato Sandwich

Cooking Time: 3 minutes

Servings: 4

Ingredients:
- 1 box Medifast Cream of Tomato Soup (1 fueling)
- 1/4 cup egg beaters (lean 1/8 or .125)
- 1 slice 2% Reduced American Fat Cheese (1/5 or .20 lean)

Directions:
1. Combine soup and egg beaters.
2. Pour uniformly over a sandwich maker's 4 squares. 3 minutes to cook.
3. Then split in half, and add cheese.
4. Experience!

100) Faux Fried Zucchini

Cooking Time: 15 minutes

Servings: 3

Ingredients:
- 1 Medifast Cream of Broccoli Soup (1 meal)
- 1 1/2 cup of zucchini, with thin slices (3 greens)
- 2 tsp. of olive oil (2 wholesome fats)
- 1/4 tsp. black pepper (1/2 seasoning)
- 1/4 tsp. garlic powder (1 seasoning)

Directions:
1. Preheat the oven to 400 ° F.
2. Slices of zucchini coat in olive oil.
3. Combine the soup and spices into a gallon Ziploc container.
4. Toss slices of zucchini in and shake to dust.
5. Marinate in the refrigerator for 10 minutes.
6. Coat a baking sheet with nonstick spray and spread the zucchini in a single layer.
7. Bake for 12 minutes, or till the edges are brown.
8. Flip slices over, broil for 3 minutes, or until browned evenly.

101) Chocolate Mint Soft Serve Brownie Bottoms

Cooking Time: 3 minutes

Serving: 10

Ingredients:
- 1 Medifast or Optavia Brownie Blend (1 fueling)
- 1 Medifast or Optavia Soft Serve Chocolate Mint Mix (1 fueling)
- 1/2 cup + 3 tbsp. of water

Directions:
1. Sprinkle with a cooking spray on two ramekins.
2. Mix brownie with 3 tablespoons of water and split into two prepared dishes. Microwave for 50 seconds, or until done. Set aside, and let it cool.
3. Mix the soft serve in a shaker jar with 1/2 cup sugar. Pour the mixture over the two brownies and uniformly divide.
4. Freeze an hour.

102) Slutty Brownie

Cooking Time: 3 minutes

Servings: 4

Ingredients:
- 1 MF brownie (1 fueling)
- 1 MF soft bake with chocolate chip (1 fueling)
- 1/4 cup 1% cottage cheese (1/6 leanest cheese)
- 1 tbsp. Walden Farms caramel syrup sugar-free (1/2 a condiment)

Directions:
1. Mix up your brownie mix as instructed and split between two small ramekins.
2. Mix up your soft bake as instructed, and set aside.
3. Whip the cottage cheese in a small blender with the syrup to pull out the lumps.
4. Pour the mixture of the cottage cheese over the brownie, then top with soft bake drops. Microwave for 1 minute (they're going to be underdone).
5. Eat warm or freeze for 30 minutes, then eat afterward.

103) Chocolate Chip Cakes

Cooking Time: 18 minutes

Servings: 2

Ingredients:
- 1 Optavia Brownie Packet, 1 easy bake with chocolate chips or 1 Cinnamon Cheese Swirl Cake
- 1 pack of Pancakes with Chocolate Chips or Original Pancakes
- 1/4 tsp. baking powder (1/2 condiment)
- 1/4 cup of water

Directions:
1. Preheat the oven to 350° C.
2. Combines the pancake mixes with one soft bake mix. Add baking powder and stirring water until combined.
3. Divide the batter into two brownie trays or muffin tins and bake until cooked for 18 minutes.

104) Pistachio Shake

Cooking Time: 0 minutes

Servings: 2

Ingredients:
- 1 French Vanilla Shake (1 fueling)
- 1 1/2 tsp. pistachio sugar-free pudding (1 1/2 condiment)
- 1 cup spinach (1 green)
- 1/2 cup cashew milk (1/2 condiment)
- 1/2 cup of water
- Hot cream

Directions:
1. Mix all of the ingredients in a mixer until well blended.
2. Serve.

105) Pudding Pies

Cooking Time: 12 minutes

Servings: 4

Ingredients:
- 1 Medifast Maple and Brown Sugar Oatmeal pack (any flavor may be used)
- 1 Medifast Banana Pudding Kit (any flavor can be used)
- 1 Splenda packet (1 condiment)
- 1/2 tsp. baking powder (1 condiment)

Directions:
1. Preheat the oven to 350° C.
2. Blend oatmeal, Splenda, and baking powder together.
3. Add water slowly until dough just sticks together (I used around one and a half cups of water, but that can vary).
4. Divide the dough into two rounds, and use two sprayed ramekins with Pam. Bake for 12 minutes at 350 degrees. Let cool down absolutely.
5. Mix 4 oz. of water with the banana pudding using the shaker cup. Spoon on a cup of oatmeal.
6. Refrigerate it to set for about 30 minutes.

106) Chocolate Cheesecake Shake

Cooking Time: 0 minutes

Servings: 2

Ingredients:
- 1 Medifast Netherlands Chocolate Shake pack (1 meal)
- 1/2 cup 1% cottage cheese (1/3 Lean)
- 1/2 cup of unsweetened almond or cashew milk (1/2 condiment)
- 1/2 tsp. vanilla extract (1/2 condiment)
- 1 cup of ice

Directions:
1. In a blender, add the chocolate shake mixture, cottage cheese, cashew or almond milk, vanilla extract, and ice.
2. Blend until smooth mixture.

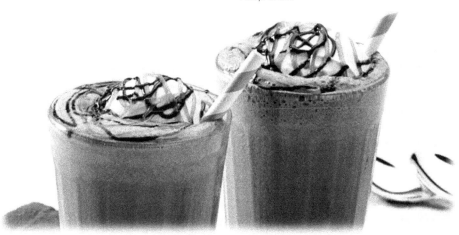

CPSIA information can be obtained
at www.ICGtesting.com
Printed in the USA
LVHW100845290121
677803LV00017B/550